D1479403
9780894643088

UNDERSTANDING PAIN: INTERPRETATION & PHILOSOPHY

UNDERSTANDING PAIN: INTERPRETATION & PHILOSOPHY

by
Mitchell T. Smolkin, M. D.

ROBERT E. KRIEGER PUBLISHING COMPANY
MALABAR, FLORIDA
1989

Original Edition 1989

Printed and Published by
ROBERT E. KRIEGER PUBLISHING CO., INC.
KRIEGER DRIVE
MALABAR, FLORIDA 32950

Library of Congress Cataloging-in-Publication Data

Smolkin, Mitchell T.
   Understanding pain : interpretation and philosophy / by Mitchell
T. Smolkin.
      p.   cm.
   Bibliography : p.
   ISBN 0-89464-308-8 (cloth)
   ISBN 0-89464-367-3 (paperback)
   1. Pain.   2. Suffering   I. Title
BJ1409.S64 1989
128'.4--dc19   88-23590
                                         CIP

10   9   8   7   6   5   4   3   2

ABSTRACT

This paper focuses on psychological suffering and its implications for philosophy. It regards bodily pain as one of the causes of suffering, others include the loss of loved ones, and the loss of (or failure to attain) social esteem, position, or property. This short work can not offer an encyclopedic coverage of all extant theories concerning the problem of pain. Confining itself mostly to Western thought, it elucidates some of the major ideas relating to its subject, discussing in some detail the widespread notion that pain carries redemptive and beneficial qualities and is therefore not truly an evil. It then describes the types of pain that seem to have no redemptive or beneficial aspects. In the final section, the paper describes responses one can make to suffering in the context of his interpretation of the meaning of pain. This section seeks to uncover flaws in certain patterns of response. Then, without attempting to offer definitive solution to the problem of pain, it suggests directions in which constructive responses to suffering may be sought.

For my wife Laura
My children Rachel and Ian
And my parents Sylvia and Samuel
Their support and understanding enrich my
life and make my achievements possible.

Table of Contents

ACKNOWLEDGMENT

I would like to thank Drs. Mitchell Aboulafia and John Gorman of the University of Houston—Clear Lake for their expert suggestions and guidance.

1

SECTION ONE: INTRODUCTION

The pleasurable life is not problematic. One tends to persist unquestioningly on his journey until he experiences pain. Severe pain elicits one's attention immediately. The unbroken revelry of the pleasant passage of time is terminated abruptly. Consciousness of the pain immediately obliterates consciousness of all else. The previously witty and articulate traveler can now only cry and groan. When the cataclysmic assault recedes enough so that consciousness again yields room for thought, it is besieged with questions: "Why did it happen? Why did it happen to me? What is the meaning of this? Is this punishment for wrong living? How can I prevent this from happening again? The sufferer who moments before was the playboy, the homecoming queen, the certified public accountant abandons these roles and becomes: The Metaphysician.

From the beginning of civilization, philosophy, religion, and literature have addressed the problem of pain and suffering.

Ancient works such as the Old Testament, the Greek Tragedies, the Bhagavad-Gita, all in their own ways deal with the reason for pain in the context of the meaning of life. With the Christian era, the central image in the consciousness of the Western world becomes that of the agony of a crucifixion. In multiple hedonistic world views, pain and its counterpart pleasure serve as the fulcrum for discussions on the meaning of life and one's proper ethical orientation to living. Leibnitz, Spinoza, and Hegel all discuss pain voluminously and hope to show, in various ways, that wrong thinking about the nature of the world makes pain the insoluble problem it seems to be. Classical social theorists like Bentham and Adam Smith use pain as a basis for explaining complex interactions of men in their societies. Contemporary writers continue the effort to find solutions to the problem of pain. Extreme skeptics may laugh at four thousand years of effort, seemingly wasted, to find meaning in pain and human life. For these thinkers who believe that the universe has no purpose, pain is as senseless and accidental as happiness, and signifies nothing. However, even they must respond in some way when they are addressed by pain. Do they change their goals and seek an easier path, or continue to assert themselves in spite of the pain? Do they capitulate or rebel?

Several issues must be discussed en route to the definition of pain this paper will employ. The first concerns the division between bodily pain and psychological suffering. Surprisingly, in an otherwise doleful topic, this issue provides the reader of the literature of pain a certain ration of humor. Like contestants in a sporting event, the writers on pain debate the issue of whether physical pain or inner anguish is the more crucial consideration in human affairs. Batting first on the team with jerseys marked "Bodily Pain," we have Karl Marx, who suggests, "There is only one antidote to mental suffering, and that is physical pain."[1]

Second up, Oscar Wilde states, "God spare me physical pain, and I'll take care of the moral pain myself."[2] Then Emile Zola's Monsieur Hennebeau, batting third, concedes that the sorrow of his unfulfilled marriage would be instantly alleviated if, like the coal miners, his "empty belly were twisted with pains that made his brain reel."[3] In our day, Elaine Scarry contends that "physical pain is able to obliterate psychological content, painful, pleasurable, and neutral."[4] She writes of the pain wracked body as a "magnified body" which enlarges its claims, engulfing all other aspects of consciousness and finally eliminating them.[5] That Dr. Scarry entitled her excellent book on the subject *The Body In Pain* leaves no doubt in the reader's mind on which team she belongs.

Rollo May, swinging for the opposition, responds that "anxiety strikes at the center core of his self and his sense of value as a self, . . . it overwhelms the person's awareness of existence, blots out his sense of time, dulls the memory of the past, and erases the future." He concludes that "this is of course why anxiety is so hard to bear, and why people will choose, if they have the chance, severe physical pain which would appear to the outside observer much worse."[6] A teammate supporting this view would be the neurophysiologist and Nobel laureate Ramon y Cajal, who states, "physical pain is easily forgotten but moral chagrin lasts indefinitely."[7]

The Book of Job, for all its antiquity perhaps the most profound work on pain the world has yet known, combines psychological and physical pain to afflict its protagonist. The work, however, recognizes the distinction between the two types of pain. Satan at first wants to afflict Job with only inner pain by removing his family and possessions (Job 1:9-12). When Job still does not curse God, Satan then says, "But lay a hand on his bones and flesh, and he will surely blaspheme You to Your face"

(Job 2:5). The devil obviously believes that bodily pain will have a greater impact on Job than inner anguish. Thus we will have to put the devil on the team with Karl Marx. However, it may be argued that Job's greatest anguish results from the inner pain of his estrangement from God, and his loss of the sense that his world is comprehensible. It is obvious that the devil has only a superficial understanding of the Book of Job.

Though this debate will no doubt continue throughout time, the present paper will endorse the primacy of inner suffering. Physical pain seems important only in so far as it causes mental anguish. A soldier, injured in battle, often feels little pain if he believes his wound is reparable and that that he will soon be sent home from the front.[8] In Stephen Crane's novella, *The Red Badge of Courage,* the protagonist is quite happy with a wound that documents his triumph over fear. When a student fractures his arm in a high school football game, the transient flash of pain may, as Dr. Scarry suggests, obliterate consciousness of all other elements. However, mental content soon returns and the event frequently causes very little suffering. In fact, the "glory" that the injury provides the adolescent athlete may lead to so much secondary gain in terms of peer approval and parental solicitude that the type of anguish that leads to the restructuring of world views seldom occurs. Had the same arm been broken by a government interrogator in a Chilean prison, the suffering would be profoundly traumatic and few would be able to escape a violent change in their world ordering. It is frequently the context of bodily pain more than the intensity or duration that determines how much suffering results. The pain that causes no inner suffering is of interest to physiologists but not to most philosophers.

This paper will focus on inner suffering and its implications for philosophy. It will regard bodily pain as one of the causes of suffering, others include the loss of loved ones, and the loss of (or failure to achieve) social esteem, position, or property. This short work cannot be an encyclopedic coverage of all extant theories concerning the problem of pain. Confining itself mostly to Western thought, it will seek to elucidate some of the major ideas relating to its subject, discussing in some detail the widespread notion that pain carries redemptive and beneficial qualities, and is therefore not truly an evil. It will then discuss the types of pain that seem to have no redemptive or beneficial aspect. Lastly, the paper will discuss what responses one can make to suffering in the context of her interpretation of the meaning of pain. This section will seek to uncover flaws in certain patterns of response to pain. Furthermore, without attempting to offer the definitive solution to the problem of pain, it will suggest directions in which constructive responses to suffering may be sought.

Having specified inner suffering as the focus of this paper, one then needs to consider whether all inner suffering is the same in terms of its philosophical importance. In two respects, all pain, whatever its etiology, seems to have the same effect on sufferers. First, as suggested above, extreme suffering elicits metaphysical speculation in nearly everyone. Even the devout Job is forced by pain to examine his world-view. Even Jesus seeks understanding of God's apparent abandonment of him. As David Bakan writes, "No experience demands and insists upon interpretation in the same way. Pain forces the question of its meaning."[9] Secondly, at least in Western thought, pain tends to isolate the sufferer from most of humanity. As will be seen in the rest of this chapter, these two characteristics of pain are related. The isolating qualities of pain are instrumental in turning the sufferer toward a metaphysical re-examination of life.

Many writers have discussed the isolating characteristic of

pain. Gabriel Marcel notes, "We flee the suffering of others, avoiding those whose disease seems incurable. Thus a gulf widens between those who are happy and those who are not, and we end up feeling hatred and contempt for those who suffer."[10] Dostoevsky asks, "Suppose I, for instance, suffer intensely. Another can never know how much I suffer, because he is another and not I. And what's more, a man is rarely ready to admit another's suffering."[11] The writhing in agony of Sophocles' Philoctetes so repelled his shipmates that they abandoned him on a small island of jagged rocks, leaving him completely separated from humanity and homeland. Albert Schweitzer writes that there is a "fellowship of those who bear the mark of pain." Those outside this fellowship tend to stare at the sufferer uncomprehendingly.[12] Norman Cousins has written of the isolation which he experienced during a serious illness. He speaks of a "wall of separation between us and the world of open movement, open sounds, open expectations."[13] In Greek tragedy, the suffering protagonist typically endures the dissolution of all his relationships until he is finally alone.

In a dramatic passage of Thornton Wilder's *The Bridge of San Luis Rey*, Esteban looks down at his identical twin brother Manuel, who has been mortally injured. The two brothers have been inseparable and they are so attuned to each other's thoughts and feelings that they frequently communicate in silence. Pain, however, ruptures their closeness. Esteban gazes at his dear brother's face "trying to imagine what great pain was."

No one really wants to go into the room of the moribund cancer patient. That scene must always shatter the complacent blind refuge one has built for himself. As Susan Sontag has pointed out in her book *Illness as a Metaphor* one prefers to nurse the illusion that the sufferer somehow deserved the pain, either by having done some evil, or more popularly since Freud, because of flaws in the sufferer's psychological constitution. The worried well can assuage their own insecurity by believing that the sufferer of tuberculosis is too sensitive or the cancer patient too repressed. This technique, while often effective for the healthy, further isolates the sick, and in addition, adds a burden of guilt that they may have caused their own illness and suffering.[14]

Elaine Scarry writes that "pain engulfs the one in pain but remains unsensed by anyone else."[15]

> *Though indisputably real to the sufferer, it is, unless accompanied by visible body damage or a disease label, unreal to others. This profound ontological split [between the sufferer and all others] is a doubling of pain's annihilating power: the lack of acknowledgment and recognition (which if present could act as a form of self extension) becomes a second form of negation and recognition, the social equivalent of the physical aversiveness.*[16]

For the religious individual who suffers, there is additionally the painful feeling that he has been abandoned even by God. As Jesus suffered at Gethsemane, he saw himself as cast out and cursed. His disciples slept and did not keep him company in this dread night. However, his greatest pain was the feeling that God was inaccessible to him as he suffered. God did not answer his cries. God had forsaken him. The theologian Dorothee Solle has written that "all extreme suffering evokes the experience of being forsaken by God."[17]

This profound solitude, attested to by so many writers, can be seen as a crucial element in eliciting the urge to metaphysics. Separated from humanity and even often from God, the sufferer floats unanchored by previous roles, aspirations, and social reinforcements. Metaphysics may become the tool that the sufferer uses in the quest to re-orient himself to the whole, to re-anchor himself. If he is successful, he ends up replacing a world view that no longer works with one that does.

Although all pain is similar in its tendency to isolate the individual and to inspire questions of meaning, the various etiologies of pain cause vastly different problems for the philosopher, the observer who reflects on suffering. For the sake of simplicity in exposition, these multiple etiologies have been combined into two major divisions—pain caused by nature and pain caused by man. Each of these major divisions is in turn separated into those instances which seem "unproblematic" and those that seem "problematic". The term "unproblematic" implies that some pain seems to offer clear benefits to the sufferer or is deserved by the sufferer in some way, and therefore conflicts less with the average observer's sense of fairness in life. This type of pain causes fewer observers to ask "how come this happened to the sufferer?" "Unproblematic" pain is pain with a weaker ability to elicit metaphysical exertion. "Problematic" pain, on the other hand, is pain that cries out with metaphysical questions.

This classification scheme is admittedly arbitrary; but it does satisfy a certain intuitive sense in most people that some pain is beneficial, or at least deserved, and other pain is simply unjust. It is true that most people have a profound tendency to assume that just pain is the pain that happens to others, while unjust pain is the variety that chiefly affects themselves. However, with effort, one can elicit some consensus, in any given society, or social group, about which pain fits which category.

In the nature-unproblematic category, one finds the pain of a hand placed carelessly in a fire. The pain is just because it has been placed there to tell one tactfully, "Idiot, get your hand out of the fire." When a child is scalded by burning coffee and the idiot is the adult that dropped it, the categorization becomes more difficult in respect to the bodily pain of the child but not in regard to the inner suffering of the adult. The lung cancer victim who smokes cigarettes may fall into the first category, if one believes he had the free will to desist from the habit. The ski jumper who lands on his head is also unproblematic, even at times amusing, since gravity is often quite helpful, is always impartial, and is part of the constant array of ground rules that nature has given people. No one asked the skier to try to fly. Pain from nature is generally unproblematic when its function is to warn us of danger, or when it proceeds as an effect from the natural laws that enable life to maintain the certain predictable consistency on which people depend. One might protest that a system of bells or whistles might be a less harsh way of warning the endangered individual than the destruction of sentient tissue. However, most would agree that certain pains that nature causes are relatively unproblematic for philosophy.

In the category of unproblematic pain caused by man, one finds pain related to punishment and to self defense. Again, punishment as a philosophic problem, could occupy a major work in philosophy. As Nietzsche taught, one must endorse a questionable theory of free will to justify punishment. Nevertheless, it is likely that most humans in most societies believe that inflicting punishment on those who have committed evil is justified and unproblematic. There is debate about whether the punishment will improve the sufferer's behavior or simply exact a proper societal revenge; but, for most, punishment as a societal prerogative does not inspire metaphysics.

Nature becomes problematic when it destroys a village with a hurricane, earthquake, or plague. Are the victims being punished for their sins, or do we simply live in an uncaring, hostile universe? Are people perhaps suffering as a necessary step in the actualization of a master plan of unspeakable goodness? Did the man who got hit by a lightening bolt while putting on the thirteenth green just have a blasphemous thought? Should he have been at church or home with his family? Why him and not me? Such natural acts set the mind on fire with metaphysical speculation. Nature-against-Man has been a popular literary theme throughout the ages, and it has also provided the material for multiple religious sermons and philosophical works.

Perhaps the greatest inspiration for the metaphysician of pain is derived from the contemplation of man's inhumanity to man. In scanning centuries of slavery, oppression of women, sadistic torturing of prisoners, genocide, the mind explodes with questions. Is humanity redeemable; does it have a future? Man's nature seems to change little over recorded time, but his destructive potential enlarges prodigiously. Nature is, in fact, far less likely to end humanity than humanity is to end itself. Humanity's infliction of pain on other humans is the most problematic aspect of our study.

In summary, most pain leads to a sense of isolation and to metaphysical speculation in the sufferer who is addressed by it, but only certain types of natural and man-caused pain are perplexing and problematic for the philosopher who studies pain. Having articulated the various types of pain, one is left with a thematic decision. What is this book to be about? I have elected to narrow its focus. I am not able to explain why nature inflicts so much pain on humanity, why its tempests are so violent or its microbes frequently so deadly. I am also unable to resolve the issue of why men are so cruel to one another in a world in which there seems to be sufficient bounty for all. Such would be lofty works on the problem of Evil and the existence of purpose or God in the universe. The objective of this paper is more modest. I merely wish to explore the effects of pain on the sufferer whether the pain is problematic or unproblematic for the outside observer. I am interested in how the sufferer responds to his pain, whether pain has a meaning for him and is somehow beneficial, or whether it is wholly destructive. I will cite numerous examples from literary and philosophical works which show how the sufferer consoles himself, what he tells himself about life to make his suffering bearable, and how others attempt to console him, or at least explain his pain. From an analysis of these examples I will hopefully indicate which approaches are flawed in some way, and which show true promise for aiding humanity in its understanding of, and response to, suffering.

2

SECTION TWO: REDEMPTIVE PAIN

There is a prevalent notion in the world religious literature that struggle and suffering are necessary in order to obtain spiritual peace and beatitude. The idea that struggle must precede the attainment of mental peace, contentment and self realization continues to be apparent even in modern secular thinkers. What on first glance appears to be an application of the Protestant ethic to the process of spiritual attainment—an insistance that we are rewarded only for hard work—seems on closer reflection to permeate most world literary works which deal with the attainment of spiritual goals. What of the poor phlegmatic fool who thinks he is content but hasn't suffered enough? The literature of redemptive pain tends to denigrate this individual. This section of the paper will attempt to document and explore the issue of redemptive pain, defined here as the pain and struggle necessary to obtain spiritual or mental peace and fulfillment. It will address the similarities between various authors' concepts of the paths one must walk to attain spiritual goals.

The first thing that has been asserted here is that, at least in respect to redemptive pain, there is little difference between religious, a-religious, and even anti-religious writers. How can this be? Walter Kaufmann has written, "If one considers the history of modern philosophy from Descartes, it is surely, for good or ill, the story of an emancipation from religion."[1] Is modern philosophy emancipated, or does it persevere in bondage? Has Nietzsche killed God and freed man, or does He still abide?

The persistance of the religious in the thought of modern man is discussed by Mircea Eliade.

> To whatever degree he may have desacralized the world, the man who has made his choice in favor of a profane life never succeeds in completely doing away with religious behavior.[2] The majority of the irreligious still behave religiously, even though they are not aware of the fact, . . . modern man . . . still retains a large stock of camouflaged myths and degenerated rituals . . . which are eclipsed in the darkness of his unconscious.[3]

Albert Einstein has written that the question "what is the meaning of life" is a religious question,[4] whether asked by a priest or an atheist. "Meaning", whether thought to be given by God or chosen by the individual, requires a commitment to an objective that we believe has quintessential importance. Religious and non-religious, Eastern and Western thinkers all stress the profound importance of reaching a goal. The goals sought are different for different thinkers. The goal for Eastern seekers seems to be a spiritual state where there are no more individual goals.

Most thinkers believe that there are goals to be achieved, that effort and pain are necessary on the path, and that the achievement of appropriate goals leads to a new world view, and to spiritual contentment, fulfillment, and peace. Since one can not prove the existence and importance of the "Goal", belief in it requires faith no less for the atheist than for the priest. The attainment of a new world view related to the Goal, is a conversion experience, no less for Nietzsche than for Augustine; the previous world view is discarded as one is converted through struggle to a new one. One is redeemed from his ignorance. He is saved, enters Nirvana, contemplates the Good, becomes the Overman, the Single One, the authentic individual. Thus, religious terminology—conversion, redemption, faith—continues to seem appropriate as long as Meaning is sought in life, and, as Einstein stated, "The man who regards his own life and that of his fellow creatures as meaningless is not merely unfortunate, but almost disqualified for life."[5]

It is important now to look at different sorts of thinkers to see how redemptive pain functions in their thought. Plato is, as usual, a good place to begin. Next, we will dicuss various Christian writers including Christian existentialists, then proceed to a brief explication of oriental ideas concerning redemptive pain. Lastly, the persistence of the idea of redemptive pain in the writings of modern atheistic or areligious thinkers will be explored. This last group will include existentialists, psychologists, sociologists, and even a novelist or two.

In Plato's Allegory of the Cave, (*The Republic*), he describes the Goal, the Path, the Pain, and the resulting beatitude inherent in the conversion experience. In the ascent from the cave into the day, the initiate would experience the painful glare of the light. Someone would have to "drag him thence by force, up the rough ascent, the steep way up." He would be "distressed and furious,"[6] and work himself to the true vision of the "Good" only by slow, difficult steps. The *Symposium* also elucidates the slow stepwise progression the seeker must traverse to behold "the Beautiful".[7] For Plato, intellectual struggle is always required to attain the true Vision, the new world view that rewards the seeker with bliss. The common man, who ridicules the philosopher, sees only shadows, and can aspire to pleasures but not bliss.

The Christian writers have provided the world with an extensive and profound body of literature on redemptive pain. There is an interesting tension in these writings unique to world literature on redemptive pain. Christian theology allows no access to salvation other than through God's grace. To say that one can achieve redemption through his own works and strivings, through his own pains, is a form of blasphemy. Man is fallen and depraved, and though some men seem relatively more moral than others, all fail absolutely in avoiding sin, all require grace for redemption. Even the greatest saints of Christendom have called themselves sinners, indeed many have excoriated themselves for their sins. This admission of failure is not to be interpreted as a false humility, but as evidence that even the greatest would fail in their attempts to walk in God's path if not for His grace in forgiving what to Him must be an abomination—sin.

Despite the knowledge that human efforts toward redemption are doomed to failure, there is a consistent and powerful strain in Christian literature that men should strive with all their might, enduring frequent tribulations, to walk in the path of God, and to understand His ways. If grace is all that is needed for salvation, if human works and strivings can not achieve redemption, and if the simple believers are much loved by Him, what then is the benefit of the nights of Gethsemane that men voluntarily experience on the path to God? If the simple are saved, what additional benefit beyond salvation can possibly be achieved by painful striving. Most Christian writers assert that there is benefit in this arduous striving after God, but they also realize that they must tread carefully on this issue to avoid the false presumption that they can approach God through their unaided efforts.

St. Augustine obviously understands that struggle can't be sufficient to enter the kingdom of God, but insists that struggle is important. The simple faith of the poor and ignorant is more valuable than the hubris of the intellectual; however, life is a process of "deepening understanding." With belief alone, God remains distant and obscure to the mind. Faith demands completion in understanding.[8] Augustine bids all to seek the face of God "through reflection upon scripture and upon creation as well as through introspection into one's own mind."[9] Indeed, the story of Augustine's own conversion in his *Confessions* is one of the most dramatic accounts of the rewards of enduring redemptive pain. After years of search for truth with the Manichaeans and Neo-Platonists, he finds himself weeping under a fig tree. He asks, "how long, how long" will he have to endure the torture of waiting for a glimpse of the eternal. A small voice tells him to open the bible. He reads and is converted.[10] The conversion may take only seconds, but the effort and pain to reach that moment are prodigious. Of course, for Augustine grace itself is based on the paradigmatic symbol of Christ suffering on the cross for the redemption of all. One need never go far to find suffering and salvation linked in Christian literature.

One of the greatest works concerning redemptive pain in world literature is the *Dark Night of the Soul* by St. John of the Cross. Written in the 16th century, this work is a poetic manual of the painful path to redemption that one travels to attain "The state of the perfect, which is that of the Divine union of the soul with God."[11] St. John, of course, realizes that "however greatly the soul itself labours, it cannot actively purify itself so as to be in the least degree prepared for the Divine union of perfection of love, if God takes not its hand and purges it not in that dark fire."[12] The painful labor which the traveler performs is merely preparatory work to open himself to God, and even for those who struggle towards God the way is not assured. Not "even half of them [succeed]—why He best knows."[13] For those who travel this "narrow, dark, and terrible road" "the soul knows only suffering."[14] "Spiritual persons suffer great trials, by reason not so much of the aridities which they suffer, as of the fear which they have of being lost on the road, thinking that all spiritual blessing is over for them, and that God has abandoned them, since they find no help or pleasure in good things."[15] The traveler learns that every notion on which he placed his identity is false and must be stripped away.

> *The soul feels itself to be so impure and miserable that it believes God to be against it . . . this causes sore grief and pain . . . What gives it the most pain is that it thinks it will never be worthy and that its good things are all over for it.[16] It suffers such pain and weakness that it nearly swoons.[17] The soul feels itself to be perishing and melting away, in the presence and sight of its miseries, in a cruel spiritual death*

even as if it had been swallowed by a beast and felt itself being devoured in the darkness of its belly, suffering each anguish as was endured by Jonah in the belly of that beast of the sea. For in this sepulchre of dark death it must needs abide until the spiritual resurrection which it hopes for.[18]

From the utter depth of the abyss, after the personality has been unraveled and when the distance to God seems longer than ever before, God's light may begin to shine. St. John describes Job left

naked upon a dung-hill, abandoned and even persecuted by his friends, filled with anguish and bitterness, and the earth covered with worms. And then the Most High God, He that lifts up the poor man from the dung-hill, was pleased to come down and speak with him face to face, revealing to him the depth and heights of his wisdom, in a way that He had never done in the time of his prosperity.[19]

Job's pain enabled him to see the face of God, a sublime vision he was unable to attain in his years of prosperity. St. John asserts that

vexation makes us to understand how the soul that is empty and disencumbered, as is necessary for his Divine influence, is instructed supernaturally by God.[20] *For this night is gradually drawing the spirit away from its ordinary and common experience of things and bringing it nearer the Divine sense which is a stranger and an alien to all human ways. It seems now to the soul that it is going forth from its very self, with much affliction.*[21] *In this way, God makes it to die all that is not naturally God so that once it is stripped*

*and denuded of its former skin, He may begin to clothe it
anew.*[22a]

The soul is clothed not only with a more profound love and
nearness to God, it is also crowned with an understanding that
is "no more a human understanding, but becomes Divine
through union with the Divine."[22b] Self knowledge also emerges
from this painful process as the state of perfection "cannot exist
unless it have these two parts, which are the knowledge of God
and of oneself."[23]

For St. John of the Cross, though it is God's grace not the
pain or the work that allows the pilgrim to arrive at the end of
the journey, somehow pain is necessary. He implies that all who
seek God must be cleansed in fire on the route. Most are to be
cleansed in the afterworld, but a few traverse most of the journey
while alive.

> *Of such are they that in truth go down alive into Hell, being
> purged here on earth in the same manner as there, since this
> purgation is that which would have to be accomplished there.
> And thus the soul that passes through this either enters not
> that place at all, or tarries there but for a very short time;
> for one hour of purgation here is more profitable than are
> many there.*[24]

Thus grace itself involves an inescapable painful process either
before or after death. If St. John has difficulty envisioning how
one can approach self knowledge and unity with God without
this suffering, four hundred years later C. S. Lewis will have
this same difficulty.

C. S. Lewis, a contemporary Christian voice, explores the
problem of pain with great lucidity in his book, *The Problem of*

Pain. In many ways, he discusses pain in a broader context than either Augustine or St. John of the Cross. Their concern was mainly the purely redemptive pain involved in an individual's turning toward God. Lewis wishes to discuss all human and even animal pain. He finds the key to the problem of human pain in Adam's Fall. Paradisal man had perceived what fallen man fails to perceive, that man is God's creature and derives his essence from God.

> *This act of self-will on the part of the creature, which constitutes an utter falseness to its true creaturely position, is the only sin that can be conceived as the Fall.*[25] *What man lost by the Fall was his original specific nature.*[26] *It was the emergence of a new kind of man—a new kind of species never made by God, had sinned itself into existence.*[27] *[Human spirit] had turned from God and become its own idol, so that though it could still turn back to God, it could do so only by painful effort, and its inclination was self-ward.*[28]

Lewis emphasizes that it is not Adam's original sin which afflicts modern man, but the daily repetition of this sin of self infatuation in each individual man and woman. God could have corrected man's error miraculously, but He instead endowed man with freedom to choose between self-intoxication and God-centeredness.

Although man's recovery from a fallen state is not possible without grace, Lewis alleges that human happiness, earthly as well as eternal, depends upon working through a painful process of self surrender in the attempt to walk again in the path of God. God, as our creator, knows what will make us happy ultimately.

21

> *When we want to be something other than the thing God wants us to be, we must be wanting what, in fact, will not make us happy,*[29] *Now the proper good of a creature is to surrender itself to its creator—to enact intellectually, voluntarily, and emotionally that relationship which is given in the mere fact of its being a creature. When it does so, it is good and happy.*[30]

As Lewis sees it, Pain plays a necessary role in the redemptive process in two ways. First, it gets one's attention, leading him to reflect on the fragility and ephemeral satisfaction of merely human goals. Second, by virtue of the nature of the journey, the road away from self and toward God must be inherently and unavoidably painful.

Lewis asserts that

> *the human spirit will not even begin to try to surrender self-will as long as all seems to be well with it.*[31] *Until the evil man finds evil unmistakably present in his existence, in the form of pain, he is engulfed in his illusion.*[32] *The creature's illusion of self sufficiency must for the creature's sake be shattered.*[33] *[He admits that] pain as God's megaphone is a terrible instrument; it may lead to final unrepented rebellion. But it gives the only opportunity the bad man can have for amendment.*[34] *While what we call "our own life" remains agreeable, we will not surrender it to Him.*[35]

Seeing pain inflicted on "bad men" causes few philosophical problems, but pain afflicting the good, is deeply disturbing even if we assume that the "good" are not free of sin. Lewis concedes that it is perplexing "to see misfortune falling on decent, inoffensive, worthy people—on capable, hard working mothers of families,"[36] but he states that

> God who made these deserving people may really be right
> when he thinks that their modest prosperity and the happiness
> of their children are not enough to make them blessed: that
> all this must fall from them in the end, and that if they have
> not learned to know Him, they will be wretched. And there-
> fore He troubles them; warning them in advance of an in-
> sufficiency that one day they will have to discover.[37a]

In fact, Lewis asserts,

> this illusion of self sufficiency may be at it strongest in some
> very honest, kindly, and temperate people and on such people,
> therefore, misfortune must fall.[37b]

Lewis goes further to state that

> the real problem is not why some humble believing people
> suffer but why some do not. Our Lord Himself, it will be
> remembered, explained the salvation of those who are for-
> tunate in this world only by referring to the unsearchable
> omnipotence of God (Mark X, 27).[38]

Thus for Lewis, given that man is inherently sinful and will not re-orient his life toward God without pain, the real philosophic problem is why some men do not have pain. As a Christian, Lewis agrees that man can only be saved by grace and not by striving. However, pain seems so necessary a part of the Divine process of redemption that, for Lewis, redemption without pain is simply inexplicably miraculous.

Having asserted the point that pain rivets one's attention, and often evokes a desire to change goals in life, Lewis goes on to discuss the reason why pain is a necessary part of the turning to God.

> *In the world as we now know it, the problem is how to recover this self surrender . . . The first answer, then to the question why our cure should be painful, is that to render back the will which we have so long claimed as our own, is in itself, whenever and however it is done, a grievous pain . . . to surrender a self will inflamed and swollen with years of usurpation is a kind of death.*[39] *The full acting out of the self surrender to God, therefore, demands pain.*[40]

Turning from self infatuation to God involves a kind of painful death in which all one's previous ways of thinking must be expunged. He quotes Hebrews IX, 22, "Without the shedding of blood there is no remission," and asserts that the old Christian doctrine of being made "perfect through suffering" (Heb ii, 10) is not incredible.

There is a plausibility to this scheme of C. S. Lewis if one accepts his assumptions, if one is a believing Christian. If humanity is fallen, not only because Adam has sinned but because each individual has sinned, if sin is a abomination to a God Who knows where true happiness lies, if life is just a brief painful test on the way to a joyous eternity, then pain on a road to redemption may be understandable. To resolve the problem of pain, Lewis requires that one adopt the understanding of the Christian that life is a desperate battle of Good and Evil, so important that God gave his only son to the fray. Once that assumption is adopted, human pain becomes an unpleasant but necessary preparation for a blissful goal. Even if the reward were not eternal but only led to a feeling of joyous fulfillment in an ephemeral life, perhaps the pain would not be so perplexing.

One can somehow accept the truly redemptive pain described by Augustine or St. John of the Cross that successfully turns a man from the hollow superficial pleasures of self infatuation to the deep abiding joy of the fulfilled man who walks with God. A believing man can even justify eternal pain inflicted on the incorrigible rebel. Even for the non-believer it is appealing to envision the ultimate and quintessential human sin as self-idolatry. However, Lewis's schema still makes it hard to understand the reason for the slow painful death of a leukemic child who dies before he can deal with issues concerning the fall, or the million Jewish children murdered by the Nazis. Perhaps these children do awaken in a joyous kingdom moments after their deaths not remembering the screams of their parents, whose attention God is getting. Perhaps their transient pain is trivial in a cosmic struggle. However, these phenomena remain inexplicable because such pain seems not to carry with it the possibility of redemption.

Lewis would argue that freedom would be meaningless if God would miraculously fix all that man breaks, and manipulate nature whenever an implacable force threatened to injure a child. "Try to exclude the possibility of suffering which the order of nature and the existence of free wills involve, and you find that you have excluded life."[41] In spite of this argument, one still has difficulty understanding the types of pain that seem not to be associated with the process of redemption. This issue will be addressed more fully later in this book. For the moment, it will be instructive to explore the ways in which Christian existentialists deal with issues of redemption and pain.

It is not too surprising to find the Christian existentialist Kierkegaard recruiting pain and renunciation as an essential companion of the road to salvation. In *Fear and Trembling*, the Knight of Resignation represents a preparatory stage in the ascent to the God-bound Knight of Faith. This knight has "drained the cup of life's profound sadness,[42] . . . and senses the pain of renouncing everything." He endures the "horrible deamon, more dreadful than death"[43] to ready himself, as the Single One, for the reception by God's grace. Though to live in truth requires constant striving for Kierkegaard, the "great man", whose faith allows him to live by virtue of the absurd, may "live joyfully and happily" every instant.

In his book *Sickness Unto Death,* Kierkegaard continues to delve into the experience of despair and discusses its necessity not only to achieve redemption, but even to become a self. "A self must be broken in order to become a self"[44] . . . "In despair . . . there is now a mounting consciousness of the self."[45] For Kierkegaard all men live in a state of despair, but most men continually deny this state. Whenever the average man senses this despair, he tends to attribute it to an external disappointment which he hopes will soon pass away. Then he can return to his life "where he left off; he had no self, and a self he did not become."[46] Without recognizing his state of despair,

> *a man does not recognize his self, he recognizes himself only by his dress . . . he recognizes that he has a self only by externals. There is no more ludicrous confusion, for a self is just infinitely different from externals.*[47]

One must confront the despair that forms the backdrop of his existence. Without this confrontation, not only is a man ignorant of his uniqueness but redemption is impossible.

> *The despairing man who is unconscious of being in despair is merely a negative step further from truth and salva-*

tion . . . to reach truth one must pierce through every nega-
tivity. . . . If repentance were to emerge, one would first have
to despair completely, to despair out and out, and then the
spirit life may break through from the very bottom.[48]

An even more direct statement on the need for suffering in
the process of redemption comes in Kierkegaard's *The Attack
Upon "Christendom."* There he states that

the fact of having suffered in the world for the truth is one
of the requisites for becoming eternally blessed. . . . For Him,
thou canst love only by suffering, or, if thou lovest Him as
He would be loved, thou wilt have suffering. Remember, one
lives only once. If that is let slip, if thou hast experienced
no suffering, if thou hast shirked it—it is eternally irre-
mediable.[49]

Kierkegaard criticizes men who regard suffering as an evil which
they try to avoid in every way. One must "relate oneself rightly
by suffering to eternity."[50] In all these writings, Kierkegaard
makes it quite clear that pain must be embraced as the only road
that will bring a man to self knowledge and salvation.

Gabriel Marcel, a Christian existentialist from the Catholic
rather than Kierkegaard's Lutheran tradition, also discusses the
need to endure pain in order to perceive

the heart of reality. . . . Those pure parts of oneself which
alone can make contact with Being are concealed from the
outset by a mass of accretions and encrustations; it is only
through a long and painful task of cleansing, or more ac-
curately, of purification, and by a painful self discipline,
that we succeed in ridding ourselves of them.[51]

Marcel implores the reader to face the suffering that is inherent in life. He writes, "whoever refuses to confront unblinkingly the necessity of suffering is nursing illusions."[52] He criticizes as flawed the secularist's hope that when politics and medicine are perfected, suffering will be avoidable. For Marcel, suffering is inevitable and constitutes an ultimate situation that can reveal Being to a man.

> *If happiness was the last word in life, possible existence would remain dormant . . . Happiness seems to threaten our true Being. . . . My suffering ceases to be a contingent fate and the sign, as it were, of my dereliction, and instead reveals existence to me.*[53]

Marcel accepts the need of Grace for redemption; however, he asserts that pain is required to open Being for each individual.

Eastern religious thought also propounds a notion of redemptive pain. The exertions of the Buddha in his search for enlightenment are instructive. He ate so little that "when I thought I would touch the skin of my stomach, I actually took hold of my spine."[54] He clenched his teeth, and held his breath until "sweat poured from my armpits . . . [and] my head felt crushed."[55] Though he later rejected asceticism as futile, he continued a rigorous program of raja yoga. His night of enlightenment was characterized by an heroic battle with the temptress Mara who assailed him with hurricanes, torrential rains, and showers of flaming rocks.[56] Buddha said, "those who follow the way might well follow the example of an ox that marches through the deep mire carrying a heavy load."[57] Even today, the

Zen initiate is given a rigorous path to follow. In being compelled to seek answers for paradoxical questions, he is reduced to the frantic condition of desperation. Ideally, he escapes from his distress into a state of enlightenment in which his thinking has left its conventional channels and the world can be seen in a new supra-rational light. Mircea Eliade has described the use in many religions of techniques designed to cause disintegration of the personality, even insanity, as a prelude to a rebirth and altered world view.[58]

The rigor of "the way" is exemplified by the statement of a Zen master that out of nine hundred aspirants he had trained, only four had become fellow masters.[59] Hinduism also has its difficult road to enlightenment and infinite Being through programs of Jnana Yoga, Bhakti Yoga, Karma Yoga, and Raja Yoga. When the goal of adepts is obtained, "nothing disrupts their peace of mind. They feel no lack, no misery, no fear, and find no cause for strife or grief. They seem always to be in good spirits, agreeable, even gay."[60] The road to this bliss in the East, however, is also strewn with thorns.

It seems reasonable to tolerate and even welcome earthly pain when eternal salvation or Nirvana is the reward. Thus, for avowed religious thinkers and Plato, a pagan who believed in immortality[61], the acceptance of redemptive pain seems reasonable. After Nietzsche killed God and denounced traditional concepts of immortality, however, the need for redemptive pain became obscure. One would predict that new atheistic writers would teach that the need for redemptive pain was now an anachronism. Though effort might still be expended to assure survival and obtain pleasure, the excess baggage of concern for redemption would fade away with the priests and other spiritual taskmasters. So many of the atheist writers surprise us, however.

They call for more pain and more concern for right living. They reintroduce sin, and continue to heap abuse on the sinners. What are the rules for this new religion, and how did we miss such a promising opportunity to rid ourselves of redemptive pain?

When Nietzsche killed God, all the fun-loving men on earth breathed a sigh of relief. Before the Divine demise, their revels of pleasure were accompanied by a nagging sense of guilt and the fear of hell fires. Now these impediments to orgy were removed. Their relief was short-lived, however. Nietzsche himself reintroduced stringent requirements for living. One now had to "live dangerously! Build [his] cities under Vesuvius. Send [his] ships into uncharted seas. Live at war with [his] peers and [himself]."[62] One must strive to become the Overman. "Man is a rope tied between beast and Overman—a rope over an abyss. A dangerous across, a dangerous on-the-way . . ."[63] One must live as if his every action represented his Truth as an individual, as if every action was to repeat itself eternally. Why do we tolerate such pain, what is our goal when it is not Heaven or God? In fact, Nietzsche is vague about the good end to be accomplished when the overman actualizes himself. One is to sacrifice himself "for the earth, that the earth may some day become the Overman's."[64] Or, more importantly for Nietzsche, one must suffer and strive because without this, man fails to achieve Being, to speak his unique truth into the void. He fails to be man, and instead lives like a beast, a "shy deer."

Thus, the Goal is to achieve Being and Truth, and to carve out a new self-determined meaning for man. Sin is redefined as the absence of striving, becoming lost among the self-satisfied masses of society. There is even a form of peace and beatitude awaiting the Overman, although his striving never ceases. The Overman becomes a man "characterized by cheerfulness, patience, unpretentiousness." Such men "have achieved the secret of the greatest fruitfulness and the greatest enjoyment of existence."[65] Thus Nietzsche describes redemptive pain, a vague goal, and a form of sin and salvation. Has God died, or do we simply worship at a new altar?

For Heidegger, the goal is to experience (our) Being and open ourselves to our possibilities. To attain this goal, one must endure the anxiety and dread of "being held out into the Nothing,"[66] as he slips away from the whole. This experience of dread changes one's world-view and as such is a conversion experience. If one turns away from his individuality and the recognition of his mortality, then one "sins", becoming inauthentic and ensnared in life, hopelessly trapped in the "public superficialities of existence."[67] Heidegger never promises bliss, but he holds that in order to experience Being at all, one must confront Death and Nothing alone and with dread. Those who do not endure this redemptive pain are lost in the crowd. They never exist.

For Sartre, the goal is similar—authentic existence lived in the knowledge and acceptance of freedom. The denial of a continually existing freedom to redesign one's life is bad faith, sin. To accept freedom and to truly exist exposes us to "anguish, vertigo, horror of the precipice."[68] Here again, redemptive pain changes our world view, avoids sin and rewards us with Authenticity, unfortunately, not bliss. By killing God, the philosophers seem to have eliminated bliss, while retaining pain and sin. They offer us Being instead of Bliss.

The existentialist philosophies and their religious language have also permeated modern psychological literature. For Abraham Maslow, the goal is also authentic existence which he calls "self-actualization". The achievement of this goal does lead to bliss, along with a new world view. Echoing Nietzche's description of the Overman, Maslow states that "self-actualizing people enjoy life . . . in practically all its aspects."[69] "They are a different breed of human beings."[70] And they possess "god-like gaity."[71] In fact, he compares those who achieve this state with "the concept of god which is contained in many religions."[72] Two things seems necessary for admission to the Kingdom of the Self-Actualized. One must have his "deficiency needs" satisfied,[73] and one must also be able to embrace his redemptive pain.

> *Growth has not only rewards and pleasures but also many intrinsic pains . . . Each step forward is a step into the unfamiliar and possibly dangerous . . . It frequently means a parting and a separation, even a kind of death prior to rebirth, with consequent nostalgia, fear, loneliness, and mourning.*[74]

If one refuses to travel the road of self development, he sins, he is guilty.

> *Intrinsic guilt is the consequence of betrayal of one's own inner nature, a turning off the path to self-actualization, . . . it is good, even necessary for a person to have instrinsic guilt when he deserves to.*[75]

One cannot escape the religious imagery in Maslow's work. In fact, he is not the exception but the rule in developmental psychology. For Erik Erikson, the goal is ego integrity, won at the cost of traversing the painful conflict-ridden stages of life. Ego integrity "is a post narcissistic love of the human ego—not of the self—as an experience which conveys some world order and spiritual sense, no matter how dearly paid for."[76] Peace comes with this new world-view, though if the stages are not well traversed, the individual ends in despair. Daniel Levinson, in his detailed study of adult development also writes of enduring stages of conflict, uncertainty, and pain, by which one might reach a plane characterized by "dignity, wisdom, authority, and creativity."[77] Redemptive pain remains necessary for these psychologists. Most humans are no longer neurotic, they are merely having growing pains. And pains are a good sign—Maslow states that "sickness might consist of not having symptoms when you should."[78]

Even secular novels and essays suggest that completing the journey of redemptive pain leads to a life of spiritual peace. In Doris Lessings's *The Golden Notebook*, Anna says to Saul:

> *What about all those marvelous people we know, aged about fifty or sixty? Well, there are a few of them . . . marvelous, mature, wise people. Real people, the phrase is, radiating serenity. And how did they get to be that way? Well, we know, don't we? Every bloody one of them's got a history of emotional crime, oh the sad bleeding corpses that litter the road to maturity of the wise, serene man or woman of fifty-odd! You simply don't get to be wise, mature, etc., unless you've been a raving cannibal for thirty years or so.*[79]

In Camus' "The Myth of Sisyphus," after his night of Gethsemane, Sisyphus is "happy".[80] Susan Sontag, in her book, *Illness as a Metaphor* goes so far as to suggest that generalized pain and suffering may even be able to redeem a society. In this book, she discusses the idea that a deficiency of suffering is bad for the culture of a society and quotes one critic who suggests that the decline of tuberculosis is partially responsible for the poor quality of contemporary art and literature.[81] There is also the popular idea that Switzerland has produced so few gifted artists because it lacks a history of tragedy and suffering. Contemporary writing abounds with images of pain leading to coveted goals.

What of the common man in all of this—the "crowd", "the shy deer", "the cattle"? What of the man who refuses to separate himself from other beings, refuses to secrete "Nothing" around himself, refuses to eschew inauthenticity and bad faith, refuses to commit his entire being to the meaning he has chosen, and seek self-actualization? For the existentialist thinker there is no question but that this common man has sinned. If he has not chosen the life of anxiety, forlorness, dizziness, fear and trembling, of sickness unto death, in short, the path of redemptive pain, he is deficient. What is this pain that has been elevated to a status as key to the promised land? Does it represent merely the wishful thinking of a neurotic who wishes to console his anguished soul by feeling superior to men who seem happier? What shall we do to help the poor souls who follow this road to meaning, who endure the redemptive pain, but who never find the bliss—instead dying after frustrated, bitter, and broken lives? What shall we do with the casualties on the road to the Overman, to authenticity, to self-actualization?

Such issues will be further discussed in Section Four of this book, but it is clear that one needs to better define the goal toward which these thinkers are so desperately striving. What is the importance of the Overman and what good for the world will really be obtained when his goal is realized? In the absence of an answer, one is left with the secondary question: why strive? To paraphrase Heidegger, why is there some meaning, and not no meaning? It is important to seek answers for these questions so that inconsistency may be avoided and men may have a clearer vision of their goals and the reasons they strive toward them. Do we strive toward self-actualization and the Overman because it feels good when we get there, or is there a sense in the writings of these thinkers that the world would be improved or redeemed if everyone strived? What is the nature of the bliss that comes as a by-product when we seek the goal? Maslow states that he has found self-actualization only in older people.[82] Have they obtained bliss through redemptive pain, or have their hormones merely decreased with increasing age and approaching senility so that they are simply not as haunted as they once were? Is the common man merely less afflicted with these hormones initially, knowing no pain, and therefore, having no incentive to strive for a new world-view?

There is a hypnosis technique in which the hypnotist induces confusion in the mind of the subject, who then escapes mental tension by going into a trance, much as enlightenment comes to the Zen initiate after wrestling with paradoxes. Is Bliss merely a physiological trick that allows us escape the unbearable? As to the common man, are we to continue to view him with contempt; or like Spinoza, can we grant him the title of "the faithful" if he practices justice and charity?[83]

Finding answers for these myriad questions is beyond the scope of this paper and the wisdom of its author. What is proposed as a future task is that "redemptive pain thinkers" form a clearer understanding of the goal they hope to achieve, and that they elucidate the value and proper uses of the anguish they invite others to embrace. Is redemptive pain necessary or merely a burdensome anachronism from which they cannot free their thoughts?

The purpose of this section of the book is not to ridicule and denigrate the frequently profound and often sublime writings of the post God-is-dead group of thinkers. Their struggles in-dicate that the search for meaning and the belief in some form of salvation for humans remains the noblest calling for any

thinker. This section merely means to challenge the view that a
new age has come, that "we have unchained this earth from its
sun."[84] Clearly these thinkers are still very much ensnared in
old problems and patterns of thought. Those who have killed
God continue to seek and create meaning. To be sure, they have
dealt a blow to organized religion, and placed the burden of
finding or choosing meaning on each individual; however, they
have not repudiated those elements which seem to form a permanent infrastructure for a life of religion and spiritual seeking.
God need not be unhappy. These secular atheistic religionists
continue to eschew the idols of the masses. They continue to
stress a life lived in commitment and faith to goals beyond the
pale of proof. They continue to realize that the spiritual road
to these goals is beset with obstacles and that one must have
courage to endure the redemptive pain of such journeying. Martin Buber writes,

> Man's three-fold living relation is first his relation to the
> world and things, second, his relation to men . . . , third, his
> relation to the mystery of being . . . which the philosopher
> calls the Absolute, and the believer calls God, and which
> cannot, in fact, be eliminated from the situation even by a
> man who rejects both designations.[85]

Thus there remains a vague, formless, churchless religion devoid of ritual. Thinkers continue to strive toward a nameless
Goal, Good, or God. They still practice metaphysics, and they
are still, in a sense, religious, the atheist no less than Augustine.
Those who believe in meaning, and strive to give their lives
meaning, still form an unbroken chain of the spirit that stretches
back through time. Rather then trying to break that chain to the
spiritual past, they might ascertain what is essential and what is

harmful to the life of Spirit, and add links into the future. They must do this because without meaning, humans will not merely be "unfortunate but almost disqualified for life."[86] The next section of the book will examine further the relation of meaning to pain.

3

SECTION THREE:
PAIN AND MEANING

Redemption is not pain's only claim to munificence. Another benefit supposedly conferred by pain is that it imbues with life and meaning, mental images that would be mere ghosts without it. In this connection, one tends to think of arcane and primitive religious practices as circumcisions, painful initiation rites, and human sacrifice. These practices obviously use pain and death to breathe life into religious symbols and events which otherwise would lack substance. One does not think of sophisticated contemporaries depending upon the injury of sensitive tissue to "flesh-out" and enliven diaphanous concepts; however, it appears that many current human activities can be viewed as later day examples of this same process. Nor is this use of pain restricted to embodying religious symbols with life. Pain continues to be used as a tool to vivify all sorts of concepts and symbols, particularly those concerning nationality, group identity, and political beliefs. It will be instructive to explore some past and present uses of pain in the process of bringing diverse ideas to life.

It would be helpful here to consider how the experience of mental imaging works phenomenally. When one reflects upon the process of imagining a tiger, one realizes that the mental image of the tiger will always be less substantial than that of a perceived tiger. The perceived tiger always has more "reality" than the imagined tiger. Except, perhaps, in dreams and certain psychotic states, the perceived tiger elicits fear that an imagined tiger is impotent to summon. The imagined tiger may only begin to stir a minimal emotional response in the imaginer. Generally, it is an advantage that men can discount the danger of imagined tigers, and run from the real ones. However, with religious symbols, and other ideas that create ultimate and abiding meaning for their believers, the ideas must have a way of coming to life. These ideas, which form the central core of a believer's life, must have even more vividness and reality than the perceived tiger. Instead of diaphanous ghosts, these core ideas and symbols must be experienced as the central reality and most substantial element of life. The god-as-mental-image must come to have more reality than oneself. The religious image created in the mind "is, in fact, described as though it instead created you. It ceases to be the offspring of the human being, and becomes the thing from which the human being himself sprung forth."[1] In practice, pain is often enlisted in the campaign to make the core images so vibrantly real.

Many authors have commented on the use of pain to enliven ideas, Elaine Scarry describes a primitive man in his attempt to enliven his image of the tree-god by inflicting pain on his hand.

> Depending on how important the tree-god is to him, he may even willfully increase the pain in his hand, . . . alterna-

40

tively, he may experience the pain as so distressful that he chooses to heal his hand and eliminate the pain, and accept the diminished vibrancy of the tree-god.[2]

The pain of this man amplifies the reality of his image.

Emile Durkheim also comments on how ritual "cruelties" are commonly executed on a particular organs or tissues in the belief that this will simulate the vitality of the religious image.[3] Bettleheim's book, *Symbolic Wounds*, lists countless painful primitive practices which serve as examples of this process. He discusses circumcisions, clitoral amputations and even ritual self inflicted mastectomies,[4] to celebrate religious ritual.

Mircea Eliade discusses in detail the use of pain in ritual. Initiation rites tend to be characterized by symbolic death and rebirth. The initiates undergo various "tortures" to symbolize this death. "The mutilations (knocking out of teeth, amputation of fingers, etc.) also carry symbolism of death . . . In addition to specific operations—such a circumcision and subincision—and to initiatory mutilations, outer external signs, such as tattooing or scarring, indicate death and resurrection."[5] In all these cases pain is a tool to make the ritual unforgettably vivid for the novitiate.

Freud makes use of pain in his theory of the evolution of human personality. Without pain, infants would remain in the primary narcissistic mode of thinking. They would be completely devoid of a sense of self. The oceanic good feeling, in which the undifferentiated world responds to one's every wish, is shattered by pain and frustration. By this means, the infant gains a sense of the other, as differentiated from himself. Freud's theory requires pain not to create religious meaning, but as the tool which makes human self-consciousness and understanding possible.

Elaine Scarry discusses the use of pain in Judeo-Christian

imagery. She writes first on the paradoxical conception of the
Hebrew God, a Being that must be acknowledged as the foun-
tainhead of reality, as the creator of all that is real, but Who
cannot be seen and can not even have an image. She comments
on the

> *incredible difficulty, the feat of imagination and agony of*
> *labor required in generating an idea of God, and holding*
> *it steadily in place (hour by hour, day by day) without any*
> *graphic image to assist the would-be believer.*[6]

Scarry then describes the biblical panorama of the dead and
wounded bodies of sinners. The multiple scenes of wounding
carry "emphatic assurance about the 'realness of God.'" "Apart
from the human body," she argues,

> *God himself has no material reality except for the countless*
> *weapons that he exists on the invisible and disembodied side*
> *of. . . . The infliction of hurt is explicitly presented as a*
> *"sign" of God's realness and therefore a solution to the prob-*
> *lem of his fictiveness.*[7a]

Suffering

> *becomes the vehicle of verification; doubt is eliminated; the*
> *incontestable reality of the sensory world becomes the incon-*
> *testable reality of a world invisible and unable to be*
> *touched.*[7b]

In Christianity, God becomes embodied in Jesus. The nar-
rative of the New Testament builds to the quintessential climax
in which horrible suffering and revelatory meaning are so com-

mingled as to be inseparable in the collective consciousness of Western man for two thousand years. The hackneyed phrase, "we all have our crosses to bear," reflects the consciousness that it is our burdens and pains that help determine one's meaningful roles in life.

Authors like Eliade and Scarry insist that pain continues to be used as a major tool to animate concepts and images. Eliade describes trivial examples in contemporary life which duplicate the painful ordeals of initiation rites.[8] In this category, one can think of basic training in the military, medical internship, and fraternity inductions. In these ordeals, the initiate experiences more pain than is strictly necessary merely to learn the tasks of his new role. The excess of pain is used to engender fear and awe for the sanctity of the group the novice is entering. Modern psychoanalysis "resembles initiatory descents into hell, the realm of ghosts, and combat with monsters"[9] in order to reestablish meaning in a stale life.

Elaine Scarry believes that war is an activity which exists primarily to verify the truth of one of two conflicting versions of reality.[10] Initially, the two potential combatants articulate different images of reality—verbal issues such as freedom, national sovereignty, the right to a disputed ground, or the extra-territorial authority of a particular ideology. War is a "contest" in which bodies and voice are juxtaposed. The goal of the contest is to out-injure the opponent until one image of reality is renounced and the other image becomes accepted reality. The body counts of recent wars help serve as a rough estimate of whose reality is winning. Some contestants are obviously willing to pay much more for their reality than other contestants, so it is not necessarily true that the victor is the party less injured. It is true, however that the victor is able to assert its reality in a manner that is no longer contested by the vanquished. The vanquished side must reconstruct its self image in a manner which accommodates this new reality. Scarry writes that "in war, the national self-definitions of the disputing countries have collided, and the dispute disappears if at least one of them agrees to retract, relinquish, or alter its own form of self belief, its own form of self extension."[11] Here too dead and injured bodies function as abiding material evidence that the contest between realities had been definitely settled. The fifty million deaths of World War II confirmed that the recognized reality in Europe after 1945 would not be that of the Nazis. War "provides by its massive opening of human bodies, a way of reconnecting the derealized and disembodied beliefs with the force and power of the material world."[12]

In fact, Scarry's entire book, *The Body in Pain*, is a brilliant discussion of the interconnectedness between pain and meaning. Her persuasive argument denies the contention that only man's primitive past required wounded bodies to animate beliefs. She implies the word still must be made flesh, and pain is the tool most frequently chosen. Man, who continues to need meaning in his life, must seek other tools in order to vivify religious and secular symbols.

4

SECTION FOUR: PAIN AS WHOLLY DESTRUCTIVE

owed by the weight of centuries he leans
Upon his hoe and gazes on the ground,
The emptiness of ages in his face,
And on his back the burden of the world.

Who made him dead to rapture and despair,
A thing that grieves not and that never hopes,
Stolid and stunned, a brother to the ox? . . .
Whose breath blew out the light within this
brain?[1]

Edwin Markham's "Man With the Hoe" is not redeemed by pain. His life is not imbued with meaning. In fact, his pain destroys him. The monotonous suffering of the day to day extinguishes his fire. Bereft of hope, lacking even the spirit to cry, he stands stunned and mute. Probably he will never recover. He is lost.

It is not the intention of this section to catalogue the unending human procession of broken bodies and tortured souls besmirching the long history of humanity. No writer would have the endurance for such a work, which would be read only by devout masochists or academicians. The intention of the section is, rather, two-fold. First, it will offer several examples to refute the contention that pain is necessarily redemptive or meaningful, offering instead, the view that pain can be wholly destructive. Second, it will present a phenomenological portrait of humans who have been destroyed by pain, hoping to provide some insight into their unique and frightening world-view.

Viktor Frankl provides a description of such a lost soul whom he observed while both were inmates of a German concentration camp. He writes:

> The prisoner who had lost faith in the future—his future—was doomed. With his loss of belief in the future, he also lost his spiritual hold; he let himself decline and became subject to mental and physical decay. Usually this happened quite suddenly, in the form of a crisis, the symptoms of which were familiar to the experienced camp inmate . . . Usually it began with the prisoner refusing to get dressed and wash, or to go out on the parade grounds. No entreaties, no blows, no threats had any effect. He just lay there, hardly moving . . . He simply gave up. There he remained, lying in his own excreta, and nothing bothered him any more.[2]

Elie Wiesel has also commented on the stunned camp survivor. "Anyone who has seen what they have seen cannot be like the others, cannot laugh, love, pray, bargain, suffer, have fun, or forget. [They have been] amputated, [not of their limbs but of] their will and their taste for life."[3]

Another description of lost souls is provided by writers in the newest subspecialty of psychiatry—care for torture victims. Since it is estimated that the governments of one third of the countries on earth use torture for political ends,[4] this is a current growth area in medicine. These experts have coined the term "torture syndrome" to describe the plight of their patients: "The victims tire easily, are unable to concentrate, and think constantly of their torture. Some believe that their tormentors are still pursuing them; others experience a constant, formless fear . . . Many victims are so disturbed that they show little interest in their children."[5] These patients are so impaired by their experience that the physicians must devise unique methods even to accomplish a physical examination. Wireless methods of obtaining electrocardiograms must be used before victims of electroshock torture can tolerate the test without panic. Dental work is often impossible in victims who had teeth drilled as part of their torture. Kitchen utensils, which before the torture connoted the warmth and security of the hearth, now have become weapons that trigger unspeakable terror.[6] The objects of civilized humane living have been transformed into symbols of Hell. Just as the victim's language has been transformed from a device of precise articulation to a pathetic cacophony of groan and cry, so also, his sense of civilization has been unmade, deconstructed. The road back for many is too long. Failures in therapy are frequent and characterized either by suicide, or by the permanent inability of the victim to experience any pleasure in living.

The theologian Dorothee Solle comments further on this destruction of humans. She writes:

47

There are forms of suffering that reduce one to a silence in which no discourse is possible any longer, in which a person ceases reacting as a human agent. Extreme external conditions such as exist in camps where people are starving, or in destructive psychosis, are examples of such senseless suffering. It is senseless because the people affected by it no longer have any possibility of determining a course of action, of learning from their experience, or of taking measures that would change anything . . . There is pain that renders people blind and deaf . . . Everything else recedes as unessential, the person becomes totally preoccupied with his suffering.[7]

She comments further that "worldly grief can lead to death; that is, it can put people into a death-like, unconnected condition of paralysis."[8] Civil War surgeon S. W. Mitchell supports this view. He writes, "perhaps few people who are not physicians can realize the influence which long continued and unendurable pain may have upon both body and mind."[9]

Nor does it require such dramatic methods to kill a human's soul or spirit. As in the Edwin Markham poem, small continuous daily doses of pain experienced in monotonous, thankless, futile labor can kill a soul slowly. At first, an individual may suffer anguish at the perceived meaninglessness of his life. Later the anguish remits. He continues his activities, and only the perceptive few will know that, at some unheralded moment in the man's past, his flame burnt out. Redemption never came, meaning eluded him, and at least from his perspective, life was a failed effort.

Modern thinkers are well aware that life presents the possibility of permanent despair and defeat, that the battle for mean-

ing and any measure of happiness is frequently lost. Gabriel
Marcel writes,

> *I can abandon myself purely and simply to my suffering,*
> *identify myself with it, and this too is a terrible temptation.*
> *I can reconcile myself to my suffering which I proclaim to*
> *be completely meaningless; however, since it is the center of*
> *my world, the world itself, centered on something meaning-*
> *less, also becomes absolutely meaningless.*[10]

In *Sickness Unto Death*, Kierkegaard seeks redemption on a
path that leads through despair. He realizes, however, that while
on this road, "Suicide will be the danger nearest to him."[11] In
Childhood and Society, Erik Erikson pictures each of the eight
stages of human development as fraught with the possibility of
permanent failure. The final stage can be characterized by either
ego integrity or despair.[12]

The psychiatrist Eugene Minkowski also reflects on the portrait of defeat that some men paint with their lives. He writes,

> *Men were no longer perceived as individuals with their per-*
> *sonal and individual values, but became pale, distorted shad-*
> *ows moving against a backdrop of hostility . . . All the*
> *complex psychic life of human beings had disappeared; they*
> *were only schematic mannequins.*[13]

Humans obviously differ greatly in their ability to tolerate
pain. The pain that destroys some men spurs others to achievements that win for them the Nobel prize. In pharmacology, there
is a term called "therapeutic ratio". For every medicine there is
a dose that is helpful, and a dose that is toxic. The therapeutic

PAIN AS WHOLLY DESTRUCTIVE

ratio deals with the relationship of these two doses. Pain may have a therapeutic ratio that differs among individuals. Some dose of pain may be necessary for human development, for focusing one's attention, for stirring questions that may lead to a positive reorientation of one's life. But each human has a threshold beyond which pain is poison. Medications can be prescribed with such ratios in mind, but pain seemingly is distributed randomly. Many are poisoned, and for these poor souls there is no consolation, for they are dead inside.

5

SECTION FIVE:
RESPONSES TO PAIN

INTRODUCTION

When pain entirely fills the consciousness of the sufferer, even the greatest wisdom on the subject seems an unwelcome platitude. Job's comforters served him best in the days before the contentious speaking began, when they just sat with him silently. With time, however, questions colonize the troubled mind; the colony inevitably grows and demands a hearing. How does one then explain pain to the fellow human, piteously suffering? How does one urge him to respond when he is addressed by pain? Can sense be made of pain? Is it comprehensible?

The world literature on pain is voluminous. A voluminous literature on a subject usually means that much remains unknown about it. When something is thoroughly known, people cease to write about it. No one writes much today about pneumococcal pneumonia because its etiologic agent and cure are known. Contrast this with the fact that entire libraries are devoted to cancer. One day cancer may occupy only a small volume, but pain will remain as an eternal subject for reflection. Pain has been humanity's perplexing companion through the millennia. It will never forsake us.

Several explanatory and reconciling ideas from the literature of pain will now be discussed. These ideas emerged at different times in the history of humanity, but none has been successfully refuted, and all survive in the modern consciousness. Within a month's time, one can hear variations of nearly all of them used to console or at least explain pain to a sufferer. The order of presentation is not crucial except that the ideas presented first will be more superficially treated because they are, in most cases, already better known. First, we will consider the Stoic response to pain. Next, related to Stoic theory, is the idea that the key to understanding pain is found in greater knowledge of how the universe is constituted. Then the views of various theologians will be discussed, especially a group of theologians who renounce the idea that God is omnipotent. Finally, several contemporary atheists will take the floor. This will be followed by a short conclusion in which the author will indulge himself by offering a personal comment on the various theories. Some critical analysis will also be included in the discussion of each view-point.

STOICS AND THEIR COUSINS

Stoicism is one of the most widely employed gifts the Greeks and Romans ever gave to humanity. It is based on the belief that the cosmos is perfect and orderly, and that the happy, virtuous man will attempt to make his life orderly as well. Man will use reason, his defining trait, to bring himself into harmony with the cosmos. To complain against the universe because life is disappointing or painful is futile and also a sign of human ignorance. Complaints emerge because of human vanity. Individuals refuse to see that happiness comes only from living in harmony with nature. Instead, they establish vain goals of wealth, social esteem, and the possessive love of others. They define their identity not by virtue but by social position, property, and love relationships. When these goals are lost, the ignorant are shattered. They have not learned that an individual can own only his virtue, his ability to react to the vicissitudes of life with equanimity and to maintain his harmony with nature.

The Stoics remind their followers that the terms of life are clear and an exit is always available. Seneca writes, "We live among things that are destined to perish. There's no ground for resentment in all this. We've entered into a world in which these are the terms of life—if you're satisfied with that, submit to them, if you're not, get out, whatever way you please."[1] Seneca advises the wise man to consider all the misfortune that may possibly befall him, to "rehearse them in your mind: exile, torture, war, shipwreck. All the terms of our human lot should be before our eyes;" then the individual will not be overwhelmed and struck numb by the events when they occur.[2]

The Stoics also realize, unlike Job's comforters, that rewards and punishments are not dispensed in life in accordance with the merits of their recipients. Marcus Aurelius acknowledges, "Yet living and dying, honor and dishonor, pain and pleasure, riches and poverty, and so forth are equally the lot of good men and bad."[3] Random fate determines the hand each man is dealt, and a bad hand can be played with as much virtue, and therefore happiness, as four aces. Epictetus prefers a theatrical analogy, "remember that you are an actor in a play, the character of which is determined by the playwright. For this is your business, to play admirably the role assigned to you; but the selection of that role is Another's."[4] This Stoical resignation to life's misfortune finds its expression in the word literature of pain at all times and in many cultures.

Eastern thought, much of which pre-dates the writings of the Stoics, endorses many of their precepts on orientation to pain. The Buddha states that life contains little but pain and suffering, which are the products of desire. He believes that desire inevitably leads to suffering—either the suffering of satiation, or that of frustration at not achieving a goal. Buddha exhorts his followers to abandon goals and de   and to live in harmony with the cosmos. The Hindu master   ce, the Bhagavad-Gita, also supports the Stoical acceptance of the vicissitudes of life. "A serene spirit accepts pleasure and pain with an even mind, and is unmoved by either."[5] One should live, it asserts, "according to the law of his nature," for then he will be in harmony with the universe. "When a man has achieved non-attachment, self-mastery, and freedom from desire through renunciation, he reaches union with Brahman."[6] This idea is quite consistent with Stoical thought.

The thought of Schopenhauer provides an interesting contrast to that of the Stoics. This nineteenth century philosopher endorses none of the assumptions of the stoics, but concludes his speculations by recommending a similar code of conduct. Schopenhauer denies that life is governed by a perfect rational cosmos. He argues, in fact, that the world is energized by "The Will" (a blind ungovernable and destructive force) and that the world ought not to exist, "that its non-existence would be preferable to its existence."[7] He believes that the pain of life far outstrips any ephemeral happiness and calls life "a business that does not cover the costs."[8] Schopenhauer rejects any attempt to rationalize or justify human suffering. These attempts he derides as "not merely an absurd, but also a really wicked way of thinking, a bitter mockery of the unspeakable suffering of mankind."[9] For the vast majority of mankind, happiness is unobtainable, and the few apparently happy people are "rare exceptions," who like "decoy birds" are placed on earth to lure the rest of humanity into a false hope.[10] Schopenhauer does agree with the Stoics, however, that seeking earthly goals merely multiplies the unhappiness of humans. People either fail to achieve their goals, lose them after achieving them, or find their goals, once achieved, painfully disappointing. Much like the Stoics, he concludes that proper conduct consists in suppressing one's desires for worldly objects, or at least in re-directing one's "Will" to contemplation or aesthetic experience.

The Stoics believe that much human suffering is caused by ignorance of the way the universe is constituted and that if they could succeed in enlarging the knowledge and world-view of humans, they could succeed in reducing the amount of suffering in the world. This view that the key to the riddle of pain is to be found in the relation of knowledge to suffering is expressed by many thinkers. In *The Guide to the Perplexed*, Maimonides discusses the book of Job from the standpoint of knowledge and ignorance. He contends that Job was virtuous but not knowledgeable about God and his world. Job's belief in the world's disorder and in the meaninglessness and injustice of his suffering was related to Job's ignorance. Once Job's intellect developed and he "knew God with a certain knowledge, he admitted that true happiness, which is the knowledge of the Deity, is granted to all who know Him, and that a human being cannot be troubled by any or all of the misfortunes in question." This knowledge, and not "the things thought to be happiness, such as health, wealth, and children [is] the ultimate goal."[11]

For Spinoza and Hegel, it is also ignorance and wrong thinking which makes suffering seem so unjust and inexplicable. Both
men are keenly aware of the suffering which plagues humanity,
but believe that the limited self-centered perspective of the individual causes him to exaggerate the significance of his own
suffering. When creation is viewed from a larger perspective it
becomes beautiful and sublime, and suffering becomes as a
thread in a perfect tapestry. Any man can be happy to be a part
of such a magnificent tapestry. Of course, for Spinoza, finite
man never can aspire to infinite perspective, but through knowledge, he can gain sufficient vision to quiet his suffering heart.
From Spinoza's point of view, the "intellectual love of God" frees
one of the suffering that is inherent in ignorantly viewing oneself
as a discrete being. The wise man sees all of creation as a perfect
unity of Divine Being. For Hegel, individuals can attain a conception of Spirit actualizing itself through history, and this vision
may remove the sting that aggravates the suffering of any one
who believes his pain is meaningless and unjust.

Kant, whose work predates Hegel, had already rejected the
view that reason was sufficient to harmonize the stark dichotomy
between human moral wisdom, and the appearance of moral
chaos which man witnesses in God's creation. In his essay, "On
the Failure of All Philosophical Essays in Theodicy," Kant states
that our reason gives us no insight whatever into the relationship
between the world of our experience and the supreme wisdom
of God. The world is the manifestation of Divine will, but as
such, it is a sealed opaque book. Kant also refers to the Book
of Job. For Kant, the voice out of the whirlwind correctly advises
humanity that God's creation and intention are inscrutable and
include pain and suffering that from man's view point will always
appear purposeless and unjust. The basis of Job's new faith is

the honest admission of a lack of knowledge, and his resignation
to the truth that his knowledge is limited. For Maimonides, Job's
knowledge increases. Kant agrees that Job becomes more knowledgeable; however, what Job has learned is that he is ignorant.
Like Socrates, Job is wise not because he knows, but because,
unlike others, he is aware of his lack of knowledge. Job learns
to abandon his egoistic concern with his personal plight; he
learns that he will never understand God's way; and lastly, he
learns to accept the advice of chapter twenty-eight—that man's
duty and happiness lies in "fearing the Lord and departing from
evil," not in profound knowledge of the cosmos.

Despite the widespread appeal of the Stoic outlook on suffering, that approach to life has its critics. As we have noted, Kant
would criticize the Stoics and other thinkers, like Spinoza and
Hegel, who believe that they can know how the universe is constituted. According to Kant, one can only see the world through
the filter of human consciousness. To stand outside one's consciousness and see the universe-in-itself is impossible. Here he
would criticize both the basic assumptions of the Stoics and those
of later thinkers who believed God had enabled them to achieve
"true" knowledge of the cosmos. Since these thinkers assume
that suffering can be ameliorated by knowledge of the universe,
the criticism that this knowledge is impossible would cast doubt
on their entire enterprise.

A second criticism of the Stoic viewpoint is that it tends to
encourage acceptance of suffering and resignation to life at
times when refusal and resistance would be more productive.
Many of the Stoics did emphasize the performance of civic duties
and efforts to improve the society; however, the basic thrust of
Stoicism is to accept one's role in the world and not to try and
change it. In the Middle ages, the Church used the Stoic ideal

to suppress any desire for progressive change arising in the populace. The ideal man for the medieval Church is the stoical "senex sapiens", the wise old man, who maintains his tranquillity and happiness independent of outer circumstances.[12] Christ is portrayed as a figure who teaches non-resistance to Caesar, and who does not physically resist his death sentence.

With the followers of Hegel, the matter is more complex. The "right-wing" Hegelians also teach that complaining about one's position in a constantly evolving world history is a sign of ignorance and selfishness. The ideal right-wing Hegelian contents himself with his position in history. The "left-wing" Hegelians do assert that men should be more active in bringing about the advent of the next age once the basic outline of history as the march to freedom is understood. This form of paticipatory progress, however, is also based on the assumption that man can have real knowledge of the universe, an assumption which leads to other abuses to be discussed later in the Camus section of the book. In general, excepting the left-wing Hegelians, the thinkers discussed in this section teach that tranquil acceptance of one's plight, and not frenetic activity to improve one's situation, is virtue.

The last criticism of Stoicism is that it encourages a certain death-in-life. One must practice death as Socrates says in Plato's *Phaedo*. One suppresses his Will, his life force and triumphs over his passions. The price of tranquility is an indifference to the events of life. Humans, devoid of their passions, achieve a "world conquering coldness, which moves along with a tone of resignation."[13] They defeat suffering by numbing themselves. They say "no" to their life force and desires. These critics wonder if it is not possible to endure suffering and to say "yes" to life.

Having concluded the discussion of Stoicism and its cousins, we will now consider two types of theological explanations for suffering. One type is as old as Job's comforters but persists in modern thought. The other type, though present for many centuries is being articulated with increasing fervor since World War II. The first variety represents a continuation of the Calvinistic heritage; the second we will call "limited-God" theology. John Calvin will open the discussion.

TWO THEOLOGICAL ANSWERS

And surely, O Lord, from the very chastisements which Thou hast inflicted upon us, we know that for the justest causes Thy wrath is kindled against us; for seeing Thou art a just Judge, thou afflictest not thy people when not offending. Therefore, beaten with Thy stripes, we acknowledge that we have provoked thy anger against us . . . We confess that we are worthy of [the punishment] and have merited them by our crimes.[14] *Scriptures teach us that pestilence, war, and other calamities of this kind are chastisements of God which He inflicts on our sins. . . . The nations whom Thou now smitest . . . , the individuals who are receiving Thy stripes . . . , [and] all who are bound in prison or afflicted with disease or poverty [must have sinned].*[15] *We are miserable sinners, conceived and born in guilt and sin, prone to iniquity and incapable of any good works and . . . in our depravity we make no end of transgressing Thy commandments.*[16]

These words of John Calvin express the old and durable idea that all or at least most of human suffering is related to humanity's Original Sin and to its continued propensity to sin. John Calvin continues to echo the beliefs of Job's comforters over a millenium and a half after God spoke from the whirlwind to refute the notion that humans could comprehend Divine motives. The views of C. S. Lewis, a modern proponent of this idea, are presented in some detail in section II of this book. To the modern secular mind, imbued with scientific concepts of causality, the words of Calvin seem extremely harsh and easily refuted by much evidence. However, before rejecting an idea that refuses to die, one must first milk it for any truth that it may contain.

As C. S. Lewis has noted, man is self-infatuated. His auto-idolatry and his adamant refusal to accept the fact that he has been placed on earth for a higher purpose lead to most human strife and therefore to human sorrow. It is man's running amuck on earth that leads to most suffering. Most natural disasters inflict far less suffering on humanity than that inflicted by man. The greatest natural disaster this country has ever seen killed 6,000 people at Galveston, Texas in 1900. World War II killed tens of millions. Humans are generally able to understand what the biblical God desires, but they choose to rebel and deify themselves instead of walking in the path of God. Surely, if there is a God, the antics of the human race must be an abomination to Him, a repetitious sin worthy of severe punishment. Even to a nonbeliever, the idolatry of self-infatuation must seem a basic tragic flaw in the human character that accounts for much, if not most, of human suffering. Many nonbelievers also have a vision of a beatific messianic goal that men fail to attain due to this flaw. Instead of seeking universal goals such as God's kingdom, or a secular kingdom in which the brotherhood of man is actualized, each individual is lost in the labyrinth of self-aggrandizement. The atheist Camus seems to suggest in his last novel, *The Fall*, that the source of evil and suffering lies in the heart of man himself. Clamence, the atheistic protagonist of the novel, rues his earlier life of self-infatuation and abandons the roles that made him rich and famous at the expense of others. Clamence states, "We cannot assert the innocence of anyone, whereas we can state with certainty the guilt of all. Every man testifies to the crime of all the others—that is my faith and hope."[17] But Clamence has not succeeded in redeeming himself from this evil. In admitting his guilt, and in pointing out to others their own, he again begins to feel superior to his neighbors. Expiation becomes just a nobler method for feeding his voracious ego. In an earlier Camus novel, *The Plague*, the character Tarrou states, "Each of us has the plague within him; no one on earth is free from it."[18] Thus even for a modern secular thinker, a notion similar in many respects to the idea of original Sin continues to arise as an explanation for much human suffering. It is difficult, despite Job and science, to refute the idea that humans bring much evil and pain upon themselves by engaging in behavior that violates codes of conduct they themselves acknowledge as correct. Nevertheless, the idea that the vast amount of human suffering, particularly the suffering of children, is a just Divine retribution for sin, is repugnant to many thinkers. They search for other explanations for suffering. Many religious thinkers do not want to be saddled with what the theologian Dorothee Solle describes as a "sadistic God".[19]

This issue of God's complicity in suffering is discussed by Ivan in *The Brothers Karamazov*. In Book V, chapter 4, he speaks with his deeply religious and saintlike brother Alyosha about suffering.[20] He confines himself to discussing the suffering of children, because he believes that adults have already *eaten the apple and know good and evil, and they have become like god. They go on eating it still. But children haven't eaten anything, and are innocent . . . If they too suffer horribly on earth, they must suffer for their father's sins, they must be punished for their fathers, who have eaten the apple. But that reasoning is of the other world and is incomprehensible for the heart of man.*

Ivan then describes multiple graphic episodes in which children are tortured and suffer great agonies, where they beat their "little aching hearts with their tiny fists in the dark and the cold." He questions the justice of a God who allows children to suffer even if they get their reward in heaven, and even if their suffering is part of a human journey to a redeemed world where happiness and peace are attained. "If all must suffer to pay for eternal harmony, what have children to do with it." He asks Alyosha to imagine that he is building a blueprint to attain future world harmony and bliss

but that it is essential and inevitable to torture to death only one tiny creature—that child beating its breast with its fists, for instance, in order to found that edifice on its unavenged tears. Would you consent to be the architect of those conditions? . . . And can you accept the idea that the men for whom you are building would agree to receive their happiness from the unatoned blood of a little victim? And accepting it would remain happy forever.

The suffering of children continues to be potent rebuttal for those who would explain all suffering as Divine punishment. Many other authors cite the suffering children as the symbol of inexplicable injustice in the world. In *The Plague*, after the magistrate's son dies horribly, Dr. Rieux says to the priest Paneloux, "Until my dying day I shall refuse to love a scheme of things in which children are put to torture."[21] In a gripping passage of Elie Wiesel's *Night*, the guards at a Nazi concentration camp decide to entertain themselves by hanging a child and two men in front of the inmates of the camp.

> *The men died quickly, but the struggle of the boy lasted half an hour. "Where is God? Where is He?", a man behind me asked. As the boy after a long time was still in agony on the rope, I heard the cry again, "Where is God now?" And I heard a voice within me answer, "Here he is—he is hanging here on this gallows."*[22]

Modern theologians continue to grapple with the problem of seemingly innocent people—children—suffering agony in a world supposedly ruled by a just, omnipotent, benevolent God. The twentieth century has carved deeper into the "slaughterbench of history" than any previous epoch, and it has brought the issue of the innocent suffering into sharp focus. Some defenders of God have been lead to renounce Him completely after contemplating Auschwitz and other recent atrocities. Alasdair McIntyre wrote a book called *Difficulties in Christian Belief* in 1959.[23] In this volume he wrestles with the grotesque reality of Auschwitz, and concludes that evil is not willed by God but is an unavoidable possibility if God truly grants self-determining agents the ability to exercise choices. "For God wills that men should do what they will, even if it is not what God would wish them to do."[24] By 1967, however, McIntyre is still struggling with the same problem, finding his earlier solution unsatisfactory. In a review of Ulrich Simon's *Theology of Auschwitz*, Mc-

Intyre renounces Christianity, the faith he had defended for years, and writes,

> *If there is an eternal God who stood by while Auschwitz happened and did nothing to prevent it, then do not let him set himself up before us on the Day of Judgment. Above all, let us have no Divine cant about his forgiving us our sins. It will be God who will need to be forgiven.*[25]

Rabbi Richard Rubenstein also renounced God after contemplating the suffering inflicted on a million Jewish children. He writes,

> *I have elected to accept what Camus has rightly called the courage of the absurd, the courage to live in a meaningless, purposeless cosmos rather than believe in a God who inflicts Auschwitz on his people.*[26]

Other religious thinkers do not reject God, but nevertheless stand dazed by the immense totality of suffering in the world. They admit they are confused by what Martin Buber called the "eclipse of God",[27] which makes it so difficult for modern man to make contact with a divinity seemingly so distant. Emile Fackenheim has written of the inadequacy of previous Jewish doctrines that purport to show that suffering is Divine punishment for sin. He writes, "However we twist and turn this doctrine in response to Auschwitz, it becomes a religious absurdity and even a sacrilege."[28] "A Messiah who is able to come but who at Auschwitz did not come, has become an impossibility."[29] Although Fackenheim does not renounce God, he does not offer an explanation of his absence at Auschwitz. The writer remains hurt, angry, and confused.

Elie Wiesel has his protagonist in *Gates of the Forest* angrily question an old Rabbi. He taunts the Rabbi who can continue to lead a service of worship to God after the horrors of the Holocaust. The Rabbi finally responds:

> *"So be it," he shouted. "He's guilty; do you think that I don't know it? That I have no eyes to see, no ears to hear? That my heart doesn't revolt? That I have no desire to beat my head against the wall and shout like a madman, to give rein to my sorrow and disappointment? Yes, he is guilty. He has become the ally of evil, of death, of murder, but the problem is still not solved. I ask you a question and dare you to answer: What is there left for us to do?"*[30]

Fackenheim and Wiesel do not endorse the answer of Job who becomes serene after accepting that the ways of God are beyond humanity's comprehension. Nor do they embrace the alternative strategy suggested by Job's wife, "to curse God, and die"(II:9). They prefer to remain in the painful confusion of men who admit they do not understand, but refuse to be serene with the reality of so much suffering.

Other modern theologians denounce the idea that suffering represents divine punishment for sin, but continue to assert that God is benevolent and loving. They do this by offering the seemingly radical doctrine that God is not omnipotent. This view, clearly articulated by the American "Personalist" philosopher Edgar Brightman in 1940[30a], has been echoed by several Contemporary Theologians. It is instructive to examine not only their criticism of "suffering as punishment" theology but also their conception of the interaction of their limited God with the world.

Dorothee Solle, a German theologian, has written critically of two traditional Christian explanations of suffering. The first she calls Theological Masochism, the second she denounces as Sadistic Theology. Theological Masochism is the assertion that suffering has been sent by God to punish, train, or test humans, and that it should be borne patiently and with humility. It is

> *a test, sent by God, that we are required to pass. It is considered a punishment that follows earlier sins . . . , or as a refining from which we come out purified.*[31a] *To that extent, the Christian interpretation of suffering amounts to a recommendation of masochism. Suffering is there to break our pride demonstrate our powerlessness, exploit our dependency.*[31b]

Solle suggests that

> *almost all Christian interpretations of suffering ignore the distinction between suffering that we can and cannot end. And by referring to the universality of sin, they deny the distinction . . . between the guilty and the innocent party.*[32]

She also suggests that Masochistic Theology encourages a lack of sensitivity toward those who suffer, because it views the sufferer as deserving of the pain which is sent to purify the soul.

She treats Theological Sadism even more forcefully. This theology reveres a God who is,

> *neither good nor logical but only extremely powerful. . . . The God who produces suffering and cosmic affliction becomes the glorious theme of a theology that directs our attention to the God who demands the impossible and tortures people.*[33]

The three propositions of sadistic theology are as follows: 1. God is the almighty ruler of the world and sends all suffering. 2. God is just. 3. All suffering is punishment for sin. The two propositions that God is all powerful and just, lead to the conclusion that all suffering has to be punishment for sin. Christian Masochism considers that God is loving as well as just. This leads to the slightly different conclusion that suffering exists to punish, or to test, train, or improve the sufferer. These two theologies taken together view suffering as either punishment or a gift sent by a just, loving God for its pedagogical value. Solle argues that "any attempt to look upon suffering as caused directly or indirectly by God stands in danger of regarding him as sadistic." This correlates with an understanding of suffering as a process within the Trinity whereby "one of the persons of the Trinity underwent suffering while another person of the trinity was the one who caused it. The first person of the Trinity casts out and annihilates the second."[34] Solle and other contemporary theologians (Burkle, Kushner) wish to avoid the intolerable third proposition of both Masochistic and Sadistic theologies by denying the first assertion—that God is all powerful. Solle admits that it is possible to conceive of a "combination of omnipotence with righteousness, viewed as absolute and perfectionistic making demands that by definition cannot be fulfilled." She is unable, however to conceive of combining omnipotence and perfect justice with love. She asserts that the suffering of the innocent (children) contradicts the view that God can be omnipotent, just and loving. Solle further questions this God's justice when she asserts,

> *Whoever grounds suffering in a almighty alien one who ordains everything has to face the question of the justice of this God . . . then all that remains is either total submission*

67

to God's omnipotence, together with renunciation of the question about his justice, as Job did at the last, or else rebellion against this God, and the awaiting of another deliverer.[35]

Although the assertion that God is not omnipotent may seem a pernicious modern blasphemy, it has been present in religious thought for centuries. The Zohar, an early medieval work of Jewish mysticism speaks dramatically of the self limitation of God which is called the Tzimtzum.[36] Before the creation of the universe, God withdrew into himself in order to leave room for creation, and for human groping and error, in the vacuum that was left. Only holy sparks, the Shekina, were left sprinkled through creation. It become the job of humans in partnership with the self-limited God to redeem the sparks and mend the flaw that was introduced into creation. It is also asserted that God does not abandon creation after the Fall. As Martin Buber writes, God does not leave creation

to lie in the abyss of its strugglings; after the sparks of his creative fire fall into the things, His glory itself descends to the world, enters into it, into exile, dwells in it, dwells with the troubled, the suffering creatures in the midst of their uncleanness—desiring to redeem them.[37]

God himself is in exile and suffers when the innocent suffer. As Albert Auer writes, God is always with the one who suffers."[38] In this view, the crucifixion of Christ is a true representation of God literally suffering from the evil in the world and the child hung by the Nazis in the book *Night* really is an aspect of the suffering God. However, since the child is not resurrected, Wiesel leaves the issue moot whether God has not in fact died on the gallows of Auschwitz. God wants to use people to mend the flaws in creation. As Solle writes, "God has no other hands than ours."[39]

In fact, "limited God" theologians all seem to endorse the idea that humans do need to help God, in Divine—human partnership, to finish creation. Thomas Muntzer discusses the distinction between the bitter and the honey-sweet Christ.[40] Luther's Reformation endorsed the view of the honey-sweet Christ who has already done everything for humans. Salvation is completed in Christ and any suffering and sin after Christ need only be charged to "Christ's account". Solle argues that if everything has indeed been done for us so that in His suffering and dying everything has been paid in full, then suffering after Christ is anticlimactic and meaningless. The human historical drama is over and humans have lived in a meaningless denouement ever since. Solle criticizes Luther's refusal to believe human works aid in attaining salvation. She prefers to think of human suffering extending and completing the journey that Christ began. Christ showed humans the way, but did not expect the journey to stop with him. The "bitter" Christ still urges His flock to struggle against human suffering.

An American theologian, Howard R. Burkle, also denounces the idea of God's omnipotence. He writes,

> *We must reject the assumption that God has unqualified power. This notion has intolerable implications. If God can do whatever he wishes, then he could have prevented Auschwitz. Since he did not, he must have wished for Auschwitz to happen, and if that is so, Auschwitz must be good and God must enjoy it. But if God enjoys Auschwitz, the human value system is totally subverted, cruelty is kindness, agony is pleasure, injustice is justice. Humanity is plunged into moral madness . . . [However,] if there are some things God*

69

*cannot do, and if preventing the Holocaust is one of them,
then God must not be charged with this atrocity against the
Jewish people. Not God but those who defied God's will are
culpable.*[41]

The Jewish theologian Eliezer Berkovitz writes that "God cannot as a rule intervene whenever man's use of freedom displeases
him." To do so would abolish good, evil, and man as well. The
real question is not "why is there undeserved suffering? But why
is there man?"[42] The Houston Rabbi Cahana states, "God is not
the maid, and religion is not an insurance policy."[43] God does
not clean up humanity's messes or guarantee the victory of the
more virtuous side in every or any conflict.

Burkle does acknowledge that God, as creator of the world,
has allowed evil and suffering to be a large part of that creation.

*The Holocaust occurred because God wills radical evil as a
possibility in this world, and because human beings, contrary
to God's primary intention willed to translate that perverse
possibility into actually . . . Given genuine human self-de-
termination, it is inevitable that God be involved in the evils
that flaw the world, and it is inevitable that the world be
flawed. Only this way can the world be decisively other than
God.*[44]

It is logically inconsistent to have a world of free creatures
who are unable to choose. He goes on to admit that

*since God is creator, he is not only involved in the evil of
the world but ultimately responsible for it. God is responsible
for the fact that there is a world and for the fact the world*

is the way it is. God is even responsible indirectly for the evil choice of human beings, even for the butchers of Auschwitz.[45]

He is responsible because in his wisdom he knows the likelihood of these evil choices. "In order to create just this world He becomes an accomplice in evil." God assumes this ultimate responsibility for the evil that is done and opens Himself to suffering, because "only if God endures such negativity can there be the radical increment of Being that the creation of this world brings."[46] Burkle believes that "Auschwitz is the cost God is willing to pay, and asks us to be willing to pay, for a world in which human beings are capable of participating significantly in the ongoing work of creation."[47] Burkle understands each individual must decide whether he can agree that the value of the world is sufficient to justify the suffering. The author admits to ignorance about why man was created with such a vast capacity for evil, but believes that this capacity represents the creative force that can be turned to good. Burkle also addresses the critics of his theology who assert that a limited God is an imperfect God. He replies that a God who exercises total control "regardless of the inclinations of those affected is not supreme goodness but sheer power—awesome but not deserving of worship." He asserts that

> *Divine perfection implies limitation. Being perfectly powerful, God allows rational creatures room to think and choose for themselves ... God exercises "adequate power", as Charles Hartshorne says; that is, God does for the world everything which "can be done and need be done by one universal or cosmic agent, and leaves to local agents the power and right to do as much as they can for themselves."*[48]

The final question which will be discussed concerning the "limited God" theology is that of what God actually does for a living. Is it true that whether one believes in God or not, he does not look for Him to do anything? Is God just a fellow weeper in a world symphony of tears? These theologians are unanimous in believing that God is active in the world and that he is always on the side of the innocent suffer. He can not interfere with free will, but he can, in most cases, give the sufferer the strength to bear the pain. He communicates a standard of good to people and steels them for the difficult task of working for world redemption. He is responsible for whatever love that exists between humans. For all believing Jews and many believing Christians, world history is a cosmic drama of perfecting creation. Without the strength and love of God to light the way and inspire those who strive after world salvation, the journey would be impossible. Even with God's help; however, the journey may be in doubt. Burkle admits that the problem with a God of limited power is the fear it arouses that the world may not ever be redeemed, that ultimately, the Divine-human partnership may lose the cosmic struggle. "With such a God the ancient dream of the coming kingdom of God turns into a nightmare of perpetual frustration and defeat, a veritable hell on earth."[49] For the limited God theologian, there is no way to escape the knowledge that the outcome of the battle is in doubt. Each sufferer must ultimately decide whether to affirm the totality of creation and be a force working towards goodness and love in the world, or whether to curse God and deny that the value of life is worth the pain. In the memorable image of Thomas Muntzer, "If you don't want to suffer for the sake of God, then you must become the devil's martyr."[50] Suffering that does not come to affirm life serves to strengthen the devil's kingdom.

ATHEISTIC APPROACHES

Is the value of the world sufficient to justify so much suffering? What if there is no God and life is "a tale told by an idiot, full of sound and fury signifying nothing"? What if the devil's martyrs are not really diabolical but only seeking to see the truth that reality thrusts so starkly into their field of vision. Dorothee Solle asserts that "atheism arises out of human suffering."[51] Many atheist thinkers of the twentieth century have either despaired of the search to find any meaning in suffering, or else stated categorically that the suffering in the world is an obscenity that can have no justification even if some meaning is found. Bertrand Russell and Bertolt Brecht are two twentieth century thinkers who have written much about suffering in the world, but believe the search for meaning is a fruitless endeavor. Albert Camus agrees that no meaning can be found already existing in the world, but believes that individuals should create meaning for themselves in their rebellion against the absurd human life situation.

Bertrand Russell insists that the existence of suffering be accepted, and that no energy be expended in the search for its meaning. He asserts that any worthwhile creed of living must begin with the acceptance of harsh and unpleasant truths. He writes, "the secret of happiness is to face the fact that the world is horrible, horrible, horrible . . . you must feel it deeply not brush it aside . . . and then you can start being happy again."[52] He asserts that humans are insignificant compared to the universe and denies the Stoic idea that there is a principle of justice at work in it. He implores the reader to give up any belief in cosmic justice because such a belief leads only to disappointment and anger at the universe and that this is a sterile and profitless response to suffering. Russell asserts that once an individual no longer believes that the universe exists to fulfill human aspirations and desires, or to mete out rewards and punishments in accordance with what people deserve, he can concentrate on what is attainable, and not waste his time on self pity and cosmic complaints.

Bertolt Brecht has devoted most of his life to describing the horrible suffering which is so inherent in the human condition. *Mother Courage* and other dramatic works depict human suffering and man's inhumanity to man with utter clarity. Brecht like Russell, despaired of finding meaning in pain and wrote that even seeking to understand suffering was a "bad habit" handed down from the time of metaphysical questions. He wrote, "we must break ourselves of the habit of walking toward places that cannot be reached on foot . . . thinking about problems that cannot be solved through thought."[53]

Albert Camus, the final author to be addressed in this study, cannot let this issue rest with the necessary recognition that suffering is meaningless, capricious, unjust. He asserts that there must be a human response to the absurd condition in which humanity is enmeshed. He is aware of the wisdom of the ancients, that "the acme of excess to the Greek mind was to beat the sea with rods."[54] However, he denies what Brecht and Russell have asserted, that railing against cosmic injustice is a sterile activity. Camus asserts that meaning emerges in the lives of individuals through their rebellion against life's absurdity. To endorse a religious meaning and justification for suffering is a form of self deception for Camus as it is for Russell and Brecht, but Camus is also unwilling to adopt a stoical acceptance of suffering. He hasn't the stomach to see suffering, to accept the harsh and unpleasant truths, and then to "start being happy again." For

Camus, the metaphysical questions are not dead because without metaphysics, meaning cannot be created in this cosmic vacuum. The Stoic is a man who has largely killed himself inside in order to avoid feeling the pain so acutely. Camus, like Nietzsche, wants his men supremely alive. He wants them to create meaning in a world that has none. He wants them to be rebels. It is instructive to reflect on what Camus means by rebellion against absurdity.

The tersest definition of what Camus calls "metaphysical rebellion" comes in Camus last major work, *The Rebel.* Camus writes,

> *Metaphysical rebellion is a claim . . . against the suffering of life and death and a protest against the human condition both for its incompleteness, thanks to death, and its wastefulness, thanks to evil. If a mass death sentence defines the human condition, then rebellion in one sense is its contemporary. At the same time that he rejects his mortality, the rebel refuses to recognize the power that compels him to live in this condition. The metaphysical rebel is therefore not definitely an atheist, as one might think him, but definitely a blasphemer. Quite simply, he blasphemes primarily in the name of order, denouncing God as the father of death, and as the supreme outrage.*[55]

For Camus, the absurdity of the human condition consists in the incongruity between what humans naturally desire, and the reality of the world. Humans naturally desire not to be injured and killed. They desire to understand life and to find meaning in living. They desire to feel at home in the universe. Despite these natural needs, man is confronted with a silent universe that does not answer human questions about meaning. He is surrounded by irrational destructiveness, and by the spectre of suffering and pain hurtling out of the void capriciously at human recipients with no regard for their relative merits. Man is estranged from a universe which seems so antagonistic to his natural needs. He feels homeless, in exile, a stranger in his own land. He hears his "nights and days filled always, everywhere with the eternal cry of human pain."[56] Man has been "sentenced, for an unknown crime to an indeterminate period of punishment. And while a good many people adapted themselves to confinement and carried out their humdrum lives as before, there were others who rebelled, and whose one idea was to break loose from the prison house." Like Ivan Karamozov (Bk V, Chap 4), Camus refuses to accept the idea that future goods such as Divine salvation or eternal happiness "can compensate for a single moment of human suffering,"[57] or a child's tears. Both Ivan Karamozov and Camus believe that "if evil is essential to Divine creation, then creation is unacceptable." They wish to replace "the reign of grace by the reign of justice."[58] They both assert that no good man would accept salvation on these terms. "There is no possible salvation for the man who feels real compassion," because he would side with the damned and for their sake reject eternity.[59]

What is to be gained by rebellion, what are its dangers, and how does one avoid merely "beating the sea with rods" in a nihilistic orgy? With great perceptiveness, Camus discusses these issues in *The Rebel*. He begins by outlining the entire history of nihilistic rebellion. He admits that once God is declared dead and life meaningless, there is the tendency to rebel in anger by engaging in irrational acts of violence and destruction. Andre Breton has written that the simplest surrealistic act consists "in going out in the street, revolver in hand, and shooting at random into the crowd."[60] Camus cites "the struggle between the will to be and the desire for annihilation, between the yes and the no, which we have discovered again and again at every stage of rebellion."[61] Citing numerous historical examples, he continually warns against this degeneration of rebellion into crime and murder.

Another danger of rebellion which Camus discusses is the substitution of human gods and concepts of salvation for the dead God. This error is more subtle than shooting at random into the crowd, but leads to much more killing and human suffering than the nihilist sniper. Camus criticizes "Nietzsche, at least in his theory of super-humanity, and Marx before him, with his classless society, [who] both replace The Beyond by the Later On."[62] In this respect, these thinkers have not abandoned the notion that history marches toward redemption in which some messianic goal will be realized. Camus urges moderation in the quest for distant goals. He writes, "the absolute is not attained nor, above all, created through history. Politics is not religion, or if it is, then it is nothing but the inquisition."[63] He contrasts rebellion, which he applauds with revolution which leads to murder in the name of vague future goals. "Revolution consists in loving a man who does not yet exist," and in murdering men who do exist.[64] "He who dedicates himself to this history, dedicates himself to nothing, and in his turn is nothing."[65] In *The Plague*, the character Tarrou renounces his revolutionary past. He states,

> For many years I've been ashamed, mortally ashamed of having been, even with the best intentions, even at many removes, a murderer in my turn . . . All I maintain is that on this

*earth there are pestilences and there are victims, and its up
to us, so far as possible, not to join forces with the pestilences.*[66]

Though obviously attuned to the dangers of rebellion, he insists that "these consequences are in no way due to rebellion
itself, or at least they occur to the extent that the rebel forgets
his original purpose."[67] What is the original purpose that has
been forgotten? Rebellion begins because the rebel denounces
the lack of justice in the world. He denounces the idea that the
end, whether it be the coming of the messianic age, or the revolution, or eternal bliss, justifies means which involve so much
suffering. Once injustice and suffering are denounced, man
needs to exert all his effort against injustice and in solidarity
with the sufferers in the world. Killing existing men for a questionable future good, would not be a rational method of exhibi-
ting solidarity with the sufferers. Nor would solidarity be shown
by stoical acceptance of the status quo. Camus urges his rebels
to renounce murder completely and work for justice and for a
decrease in suffering. Like Dr. Rieux in *The Plague*, one should
take the victim's side and "share with his fellow citizens the only
certitude they have in common—love, exile, suffering."[68]

What can be accomplished through rebellion? Camus' goals
are modest. He realizes that the rebel is doomed to "a never
ending defeat,"[69] in that death, finitude and suffering will always
conquer him. He realizes that after man has mastered everything
in creation that can be mastered and rectified everything that
can be rectified,

*children will still die unjustly even in a perfect society. Even
by his greatest effort man can only purpose to diminish ar-*

ithmetically the sufferings of the world. But the injustice and the suffering will remain and, no matter how limited they are, they will not cease to be an outrage.[70]

However, there are ephemeral victories and rewards for the rebel.

He who dedicates himself for the duration of his life to the house he builds, to the dignity of mankind, dedicates himself to the earth and reaps from it the harvest that sows its seed and sustains the world again and again.[71] *Those whose desires are limited to man and his humble yet formidable love, should enter, if only now and then, into their reward.*[72] *They know that if there is one thing one can always yearn for and sometimes attain, it is human love.*[73]

Society must be arranged to limit injustice and suffering as much as possible so that each individual has the leisure and freedom to pursue his own search for meaning. Future utopias must be renounced, and "history can no longer be presented as an object of worship."[74] "It is time to forsake our age and its adolescent furies," and to aim for what is possible—more justice, solidarity, and love among men. The rebel must "reject divinity in order to share in the struggles and destiny of all men."[75] Redemption is impossible. Human dignity and love can intermittently be achieved with struggle and constant vigilance against the plague bacillus that "never dies or disappears for good . . . [but can] rouse up its rats again and send them forth to die in a happy city."[76]

CONCLUSION

The problem of pain has no neat solution. There is no way to complete this modest work with a triumphant flourish and a Q.E.D. I have encountered no pithy little epithet that will serve the reader when a loved one dies, or even when a rear molar needs a root canal. No generalizations can suffice. Pain is redemptive for some: it forces a positive change in their interaction with the world, and ultimately deepens their happiness in living. For others it is wholly destructive; it mutilates their bodies and souls, and they never recover. The existentialists who urge everyone to confront his death and his pain are wrong to do so. They, of all people, should realize that every individual is unique and what is good for one may be harmful for another.

How then to offer comfort in the face of tragedy, or to explain the existence of pain to those who suffer? This section has described options that recur in the literature of pain. Some see pain as a trivial aspect of a universe of unspeakable grandeur and perfection, and can derive joy from running as a thread through such a sublime tapestry. Others opt to affirm the idea that humans are deeply flawed by self-idolatry, and that punishment will continue to be truly just, until all turn to God and are redeemed by Grace. Other groups, despite their recognition that humans are flawed by unrepentant self-infatuation, reject the spectre of a sadistic God, and embrace a self-limited God whom they envision as always "with" the sufferer. Still others adopt a stoical response to suffering, a response which may reflect a cultivated insensitivity, a partial death in life, a blunting of life's joys as well as its pains, and which may leave its advocates less caring about the pains of others. Finally, there are those who rebel, proclaiming pain to be an outrage, and spurning any explanation which attempts to justify it. They wage a war they recognize as ultimately futile against an uncaring cosmos and endeavor to establish an ephemeral oasis of human love within the vacuum of reality.

When I initiated this project, my goal was to clarify my own position with regard to the problem of pain. Sadly, my vision remains slightly myopic. However, several of the examined explanations appeal to me, and here, as author's prerogative, I have allowed myself a personal comment.

I cannot accept the view that God kills children because adults sin, nor the view that rewards in heaven compensate for suffering on earth, nor the view that the elegance of the Divine Tapestry of the universe justifies such a terrible twisting of its threads. I cannot discern the Divine Idea in History nor the oneness of all creation. I balk at any explanation that justifies pain; "justified pain" inevitably lead to an insensitivity towards the suffering of others.

I have come to accept my vacillations of disposition. On some days I am a "limited God" believer, who worships Him in a limited manner. This God suffers with the victims of pain, seeking to strengthen them in their struggle against evil. I always root for the success of this Divine-human partnership, while always recognizing that its chances for failure are immense.

On many other occasions, I am an angry atheist, and Camus becomes my "patron saint." I, too, reject ideology, renounce murder, and try to assist a suffering humanity in its futile battle against the bleakness of the universe. Happily for me, the positions of "limited God" theologists and Camus-rebels can mesh harmoniously in a campaign to expunge the world's hate and replace it with love.

To me, the most aesthetically pleasing are the views of Elie Wiesel, who God-wrestles in every work that he writes. He finds God guilty in a formal trial, but will not abandon his belief in

Him, nor will he submit to God's enemies (*Trial of God*). Wiesel lives on the razor's edge of his own paradox, shifting his weight cautiously, so that he does not fall either to one side or the other of his dilemma.

Often, too often, I simply despair of the immensity of the problem of pain, and anesthetize myself, like so many of our time, by sitting in front of a television. Most days, though, to poorly paraphrase Job (28:28), I seek to depart from evil, and I worry about God a lot.

NOTES

SECTION ONE: INTRODUCTION

1. Elaine Scarry, *The Body in Pain*, (New York: Oxford Univ. Press, 1985), p. 33.
2. Scarry, p. 33.
3. Scarry, p. 34.
4. Scarry, p. 34.
5. Scarry, p. 267.
6. Rollo May, "Contributions of Existential Psychology," in *Existence*, ed. Rollo May, Ernest Angel, and Henri F. Ellenberger, (New York: Simon and Schuster, 1958), p. 51.
7. Maurice B. Strauss, ed., *Familiar Medical Quotations*, (Boston: Little Brown and Company, 1968), p. 356.
8. David Bakan, *Disease, Pain, and Sacrifice: Toward a Psychology of Suffering*, (Chicago: The Univ. of Chicago Press, 1968), p.87.
9. Bakan, p. 57.
10. Gabriel Marcel "Creative Fidelity," in his *Creative Fidelity*, trans.

Robert Rosthal, (New York: The Crossroad Publishing Co., 1982) p. 245.

11. Fyodor Dostoyevsky, *The Brothers Karamazov*, trans. Constance Garnett, ed. Manuel Komroff, (New York: The New American Library, Inc., 1957), Bk. V, chap. 4, p. 218.

12. Norman Cousins, *Anatomy of an Illness as Perceived by the Patient*, (New York: W. W. Norton and Co., 1979), p. 153.

13. Cousins, p. 153.

14. Susan Sontag, *Illness as a Metaphor*, (New York: Vintage Books, 1979), pp. 46 and 61

15. Scarry, p. 52.

16. Scarry, p. 56.

17. Dorothy Solle, *Suffering*, trans. Everett R. Kalin, (Philadelphia: Fortress Press, 1975), p. 85.

SECTION TWO: REDEMPTIVE PAIN

1. Friedrich Nietzsche, *The Portable Nietzsche*, trans. and ed. Walter Kaufmann, (New York: Penguin Books, 1959), Intro., p. 17.

2. Mircea Eliade, *The Sacred and the Profane*, (New York: A Harvest Harcourt Brace Johanovich Book, 1959), p. 23.

3. Eliade, pp. 204 and 213

4. Albert Einstein, *The World as I See It*, (New York: Philosophical Library, Inc., 1949), p. 1.

5. Einstein, p. 1.

6. Plato, *Great Dialogues of Plato*, trans. W. H. D. Rouse, (New York: Mentor Books, The New American Library, 1956), Bk. VIII p. 313.

7. Plato, p. 69

8. R. A. Markus, "St. Augustine," in *The Encyclopedia of Phi-*

losophy, Paul Edwards, ed., (New York: Macmillan Publishing Co., Inc. and The Free Press, 1967), I, p. 199.

9. Robert Meagher, *Augustine: An Introduction*, (New York: Harper and Row, 1978), p. 262.

10. Meagher, p. 63.

11. St. John of the Cross, *Dark Night of the Soul*, 3rd. rev. ed., (New York: Image Books, 1959), Bk. I, chap. 1, p. 37.

12. St. John, Bk. I, chap. 3, p. 46.

13. St. John, Bk. I, chap. 9, p. 69.

14. St. John, Bk. I, chap. 11, p. 74.

15. St. John, Bk. I, chap. 10, p. 69.

16. St. John, Bk. II, chap. 5, p. 102.

17. St. John, Bk. II, chap. 5, p. 103.

18. St. John, Bk. II, chap. 6, p. 104.

19. St. John, Bk. I, chap. 12, p. 78.

20. St. John, Bk. I, chap. 12, p. 79.

21. St. John, Bk. II, chap. 9, p. 123.

22a and 22b. St. John, Bk. II, chap. 13, p. 146.

23. St. John, Bk. II, chap. 18, p. 165.

24. St. John, Bk. II, chap. 6, pp. 107-108.

25. C. S. Lewis, *The Problem of Pain*, (New York: Macmillan Publishing Co., Inc., 1962) p. 80

26. Lewis, p. 82.

27. Lewis, p. 83.

28. Lewis, p. 83.

29. Lewis, p. 52.

30. Lewis, p. 90.

31. Lewis, p. 92.

32. Lewis, p. 95.

33. Lewis, p. 97.

34. Lewis, p. 95.

35. Lewis, p. 96.

36. Lewis, p. 96.
37a and 37b. Lewis, pp. 97-98.
38. Lewis, p. 104.
39. Lewis, p. 91.
40. Lewis, p. 99.
41. Lewis, p. 34.
42. Soren Kierkegaard, *A Kierkegaard Anthology*, Robert Bretall, ed., (New York: Modern Library [Random House], 1946), p.121.
43. Kierkegaard, p. 128.
44. Kierkegaard, p. 364.
45. Kierkegaard, p. 366.
46. Kierkegaard, p. 353.
47. Kierkegaard, p. 353.
48. Kierkegaard, p. 346 and 359.
49. Kierkegaard, p. 459.
50. Kierkegaard, p. 459.
51. Marcel, "An Outline of a Concrete Philosophy," p. 66.
52. Marcel, "Karl Jaspers," p. 245.
53. Marcel, p. 245.
54. Smith, Huston, *The Religions of Man*, (New York: Harper and Brothers, 1958), p. 83.
55. Smith, p. 83.
56. Smith, p. 84.
57. Smith, p. 107.
58. Eliade, p. 196.
59. Smith, p. 129.
60. Smith, p. 29.
61. Plato, "Phaedo," pp. 510-518.
62. Nietzsche, "The Gay Science," p. 97.
63. Nietzsche, "Thus Spake Zarathustra," p. 126.
64. Nietzsche, p. 127.

65. Nietzsche, "The Gay Science," p. 97.
66. Martin Heidegger, "What is Metaphysics?" in *Basic Writings*, ed. David Farrell Krell, (New York: Harper and Row, 1977), p. 105.
67. Heidegger, p. 106.
68. Jean-Paul Sartre, "Being and Nothingness," in *The Philosophy of Jean-Paul Sartre*, Robert Dennon Cumming, ed., (New York: Vintage Books, 1965), pp. 116-119.
69. Abraham Maslow, *Toward a Psychology of Being*, (Princeton: D. Van Nostrand Co., Inc., 1962), p. 29.
70. Maslow, p. 67.
71. Maslow, p. 100.
72. Maslow, p. 77.
73. Maslow, p. 21.
74. Maslow, p. 190.
75. Maslow, p. 182, (my italics).
76. Erik H. Erikson, *Childhood and Society*, 2nd. ed., (New York: W. W. Norton and Co., Inc., 1962), p. 268.
77. Daniel J. Levinson, *The Seasons of a Man's Life*, (New York: Ballantine Books, 1978), p. 330.
78. Maslow, p. 7.
79. Doris Lessing, *The Golden Notebook*, (New York: Bantam Books, 1973), p. 626.
80. Albert Camus, "The Myth of Sisyphus," in *The Myth of Sisyphus and Other Essays*, trans. Justin O'Brien (New York: Vintage Books, 1955), p. 91
81. Sontag, p. 32.
82. Maslow, p. 24.
83. Benedict de Spinoza, *A Theologico-Political Treatise*, trans. R. H. M. Elwis, (New York: Dover Publications, Inc., 1951), chap. XIV, p. 186.
84. Nietzsche, "The Gay Science," p. 95.

85. Martin Buber, "What is Man?" in *Between Man and Man,* trans. Ronald Gregor Smith, (New York: The Macmillan Co., 1965), p. 177.
86. Einstein, p.1.

SECTION THREE: PAIN AND MEANING

1. Scarry, p. 205
2. Scarry, p. 148
3. Emile Durkheim, *The Elementary Forms of the Religious Life,* (Glencoe, Ill.: The Free Press, 1947), p. 314.
4. Bruno Bettelheim, *Symbolic Wounds,* rev. ed. (New York: Collier Books, 1962) p. 91.
5. Eliade, p. 190.
6. Scarry, p. 198.
7a and 7b. Scarry, pp. 200-202.
8. Eliade, p. 208.
9. Eliade, p. 208.
10. Scarry, p. 63.
11. Scarry, p. 114.
12. Scarry, p. 128.

SECTION FOUR: PAIN AS WHOLLY DESTRUCTIVE

1. Edwin Markham, "The Man with the Hoe," in *A Pocket Book of Modern Verse,* ed. Oscar Williams, rev. ed., (New York: Washington Square Press, Inc., 1958)
2. Viktor E. Frankl, *Man's Search for Meaning,* trans. Ilse Lasch, (New York: Pocket Books, 1963), pp. 117-118.

3. Elie Wiesel, *The Accident,* (New York: Avon Books, 1970), p. 79.
4. Amado Padilla and Lillian Comas-Diaz, "A State of Fear," *Psychology Today,* 20, No. 11, Nov. 1986, p. 60.
5. Kevin Krajick, "Healing Broken Minds," *Psychology Today,* 20, No. 11, Nov. 1986, p. 69.
6. Scarry, p. 41.
7. Solle, p. 68.
8. Solle, p. 134.
9. Scarry, p. 55.
10. Marcel, "An Outline of a Concrete Philosophy," in *Creative Fidelity,* p.75
11. Kierkegaard, "Sickness unto Death," in *A Kierkegaard Anthology,* p.364.
12. Erikson, p. 268.
13. Eugene Minkowski, "Findings in a Case of Schizophrenic Depression," in *Existence,* p. 135.

SECTION FIVE: RESPONSES TO PAIN

1. Seneca, *Letters From a Stoic,* trans. Robin Campbell, (Great Britain: Penguin Books, 1969), Letter XCI, pp. 181-182.
2. Seneca, Letter XCI, p.179.
3. Marcus Aurelius, *Meditations,* trans. Maxwell Staniforth, (Great Britain: Penguin Books, 1964), Bk. II, No. 11, p. 48.
4. Epictetus, "Enchiridion", in *Marcus Aurelius, Meditations and Epictetus, Enchiridion,* (Chicago: Henry Regnery Co., 1956), No. 17, p. 179.
5. *The Song of God: Bhagavad-Gita,* trans. Swami Prabhavananda and Christopher Isherwood, (New York: New American Library, 1972), chap. II, p. 36.

6. *Bhagavad-Gita,* chap. 18, p.127.
7. Arthur Schopenhauer, *The World as Will and Representation,* trans. E. F. J. Payne, (New York: Dover Publications, Inc., 1958), II, chap. XLVI, p.576.
8. Schopenhauer, II, chap. XLVI, p. 574.
9. Schopenhauer, I, Bk. IV, chap. 59, p. 326.
10. Schopenhauer, II, chap. XLVI, p. 573.
11. Nahum N. Glatzer, Ed. *The Dimensions of Job,* (New York: Schocken Books, 1969), Intro., p. 21.
12. Solle, p. 99.
13. Solle, p. 100.
14. Solle, p. 9.
15. Solle, p. 24.
16. Solle, p. 23.
17. Albert Camus, *The Fall,* trans. Justin O'Brien, (New York: Vintage Books, 1956) p. 110.
18. Albert Camus, *The Plague,* trans. Stuart Gilbert, (New York: The Modern Library, 1948) p. 229.
19. Solle, p. 26.
20. Dostoyevsky, *The Brothers Karamazov,* Bk. V, chap. 4, pp. 218-227)
21. Camus, *Plague,* p. 197.
22. Elie Wiesel, *Night,* trans. Stella Rodway, (New York: Bantam Books, 1960), pp. 61-62.
23. Alasdair McIntyre, *Difficulties in Christian Belief,* (London: SCM Press, 1959)
24. Howard R. Burkle, *God, Suffering, and Belief,* (Nashville: Abingdon, 1977) p. 18.
25. Burkle, p. 17.
26. Burkle, p. 50.
27. Martin Buber, *Eclipse of God,* (New York: Harper and Row, 1952)

28. Emil L. Fackenheim, *God's Presence in History*, (New York: Harper and Row, 1970), p. 73.

29. Fackenheim, p. 78.

30. Elie Wiesel, *The Gates of the Forest*, trans. Frances Frenaye, (New York: Avon Books, 1966), pp. 196-197.

30a. Edgar S. Brightman, *Philosophy of Religion*, (New York: Prentice-Hall, Inc., 1940), pp. 336–338.

31a and 31b. Solle, p. 19.

32. Solle, p. 19.

33. Solle, p. 22.

34. Solle, p. 27.

35. Solle, p. 134.

36. Gershom Scholem, *On the Kabbalah and its Symbolism*, trans. Ralph Manheim, (New York: Schocken Books, 1965), pp. 110-111.

37. Martin Buber, *The Origin and Meaning of Hasidism*, ed. and trans. Maurice Friedman, (New York: Horizon Press, 1960) chap. III. p. 101.

38. Solle, p. 102.

39. Solle, p. 149.

40. Solle, p. 129.

41. Burkle, pp. 52-53.

42. Eliezer Berkovitz, *Faith After the Holocaust*, (New York: KTAV, 1973), p. 105.

43. Rabbi Cahana, Kol Ami Yom Kippur Service, Houston, 1986.

44. Burkle, pp. 57-58.

45. Burkle, pp. 59-60.

46. Burkle, p. 60.

47. Burkle, p. 62.

48. Burkle, pp. 53-54.

49. Burkle, p. 118.

50. Solle, p. 133.
51. Solle, p. 143.
52. Alan Wood, *Bertrand Russell: The Passionate Sceptic*, (New York: Simon and Schuster, 1958), p. 237.
53. Solle, p. 144.
54. Albert Camus, *The Rebel*, trans. Anthony Bower, (New York: Vintage Books, 1956), p. 27.
55. Camus, *Rebel*, p. 24.
56. Camus, *Plague*, p. 37.
57. Camus, *Plague*, p. 202.
58. Camus, *Rebel*, pp. 56-57.
59. Camus, *Rebel*, p. 57.
60. Camus, *Rebel*, p. 93.
61. Camus, *Rebel*, p. 91.
62. Camus, *Rebel*, p. 79.
63. Camus, *Rebel*, p. 302.
64. Camus, *Rebel*, p. 96.
65. Camus, *Rebel*, p. 302.
66. Camus, *Plague*, p. 229.
67. Camus, *Rebel*, p. 25.
68. Camus, *Plague*, p. 272.
69. Camus, *Plague*, p. 118.
70. Camus, *Rebel*, p. 303.
71. Camus, *Rebel*, p. 302.
72. Camus, *Plague*, p. 271.
73. Camus, *Plague*, p. 271.
74. Camus, *Rebel*, p. 302.
75. Camus, *Rebel*, p. 306.
76. Camus, *Plague*, p. 278.